10662994

Now it's easy to identi... ...you eat. You can carry this ... ...guide when you do your food shopping or dine out—and make wise choices to safeguard your health!

Don't miss:

ARE EGGS BAD FOR YOU?

Recent scientific studies show that eating an egg a day is safe for most people—and safer than eating just egg whites or egg substitutes!

WHAT IS THE WORST TRANS FAT FOOD?

Doughnuts. Toaster pastries aren't far behind. And you should watch out for snack foods.

WHICH VEGETABLE OIL IS BEST?

Probably extra virgin olive oil.

WHAT'S THE BEST WAY TO AVOID FAST-FOOD FAT?

The average American eats in a fast-food restaurant twice a week. The typical meal contains 1400 calories, including 135 mg of cholesterol. Worse, there are 15 grams of trans fats in the fries. The bottom line: Avoid fast-food fat by eating somewhere else.

THE GOOD FAT, BAD FAT COUNTER

The GOOD FAT, BAD FAT *Counter*

SHEILA BUFF

St. Martin's Paperbacks

THE GOOD FAT, BAD FAT COUNTER

Copyright © 2002 by Sheila Buff.

ISBN: 0-312-98153-8

Printed in the United States of America

St. Martin's Paperbacks edition / May 2002

St. Martin's Paperbacks are published by St. Martin's Press, 175 Fifth Avenue, New York, NY 10010.

10 9 8 7 6 5 4 3

CONTENTS

Chapter One
FATS AND FATOPHOBIA

Eat less fat! You hear the message endlessly from doctors, nutritionists, and everyone else. It's repeated in every media story about diet and health, it's taught in schools, and it's been embraced by the food industry. Yet even as we're all supposedly eating less fat, more Americans are overweight—one in two adults, one in four children—than ever before. What's going on here?

The problem is that the message is too simple. We're now in the grip of fatophobia—we see all fat as bad, no matter what.

The truth about fat is far more complex. Eating fat doesn't necessarily make you fat, and not all fat is bad. In fact, there are some kinds of fat you have to have for good health. A more accurate and helpful message would be: Eat more of some kinds of fats, less of others, and avoid one kind of fat whenever possible. Sure, it's a more complicated message, but it's also one that could help save your life.

FAT FACTS

A fat is any oily, organic compound that doesn't dissolve in water (just as oil floats on top of water) but does dissolve in oil or organic solvents. Chemically speaking, a fatty acid is made from a chain of carbon and hydrogen atoms—think of them as the building blocks of fat. (Later chapters on different kinds of fat go into this in a little more detail.)

The natural fats we eat fall into three basic categories:

1. *Saturated fats.* These fats are solid at room temperature; butter, lard, and suet are good examples.

2. *Monounsaturated fats.* Liquid at room temperature, monounsaturated fats include olive oil and many nut oils.

3. *Polyunsaturated fats.* Polyunsaturated fats are also liquid at room temperature. Canola oil, safflower oil, corn oil, and many other widely used vegetable cooking oils are polyunsaturated fats. The oil found in fatty fish is also polyunsaturated.

Polyunsaturated fatty acids fall into two main groups: omega-3 fatty acids (alpha-linolenic acid) and omega-6 fatty acids (linoleic acid). These two types of oils are essential: You must have some in your diet for good health. Just as you have to get your vitamins from the food you eat, the essential oils also must come from your diet.

THE UNNATURAL FAT

The American diet today is on the low side for good fats, mostly because we eat a lot of a completely unnatural fat: trans fatty acids, or trans fat for short. Also known as partially hydrogenated vegetable oils, trans fats are vegetable oils that have been chemically modified to be more saturated.

What makes trans fat so bad? Plenty. These unnatural fats raise the level of dangerous cholesterol in your blood, causing clogged arteries and heart disease. In fact, trans fats raise your cholesterol level about twice as much as saturated fat does. Even worse, trans fats are so widely used in processed foods, fried foods, and fast foods that they're hard to avoid.

Just check the ingredients list on almost any prepared or baked good and you'll see partially hydrogenated vegetable oil somewhere on it.

The evidence against trans fat is now so convincing that the federal Food and Drug Agency (FDA) has announced plans to make food manufacturers list the amount of trans fats in their products on the food facts label. Chapter 5 explains the proposed labeling regulation and how it will help consumers avoid this deadly fat.

CHOLESTEROL CONCERNS

No discussion of dietary fat would be complete without a mention of cholesterol—even though this dreaded substance isn't really a fat at all. Cholesterol is a waxy chemical compound manufactured by your body. It's necessary for a variety of important functions, such as producing the hormones testosterone and estrogen and building cell membranes and brain and nerve tissue. Most medical authorities believe that high levels of cholesterol in the blood play a major role in causing clogged arteries and heart disease. High blood cholesterol, in turn, may be caused by eating animal foods such as meat, dairy products, and eggs, which contain cholesterol. Although this connection has yet to be fully proved, current dietary guidelines suggest that dietary cholesterol should be limited to no more than 300 milligrams a day. Chapter 4 discusses the dangers and benefits to your health of dietary cholesterol.

FATS ARE MIXTURES

It's important to remember that every fat is really a mixture of saturated, monounsaturated, and polyunsaturated fatty acids. One type of fatty acid is generally in the majority, though, and the fat is classified on that basis. Butter, for instance, is put into the saturated fat category because it contains mostly saturated fat. Butter is 81 percent fat. (The rest is mostly water.) One tablespoon (about 15 grams) contains 12.2 grams of fat, of which 7.6 grams are saturated fat, 3.6 grams are monounsaturated fat, and 0.5 grams are polyunsaturated fats. And because butter is a dairy product, it also contains 33 milligrams of cholesterol. So, a tablespoon of butter is more than half saturated fat, which is bad, but also has monounsaturated and polyunsaturated fats, which are good. And as Chapter 5 explains, think again before deciding margarine, which contains trans fats, is better for your health than butter.

It's also important to remember that every gram of fat, no matter what kind it is or where it comes from, contains 9 calories. For comparison, a gram of carbohydrates or protein contains 4 calories. Because a gram of fat contains 5 more calories than a gram of carbohydrates, in theory eating less fat means you eat fewer calories, which should in turn lead to weight loss. In practice, the opposite usually happens: To make up for the missing fat (and taste) in reduced-fat foods, manufacturers put in more sugar or other ingredients. The calories per serving don't decrease and you don't lose weight. In fact, you might gain, because you might start eating *more* calories. Why? You think that because the food has less fat, it's somehow more healthful and you can eat more of it. Also, fat in food plays an important role in satisfying your appetite and making you feel full. With less fat in your food, you don't feel as satisfied and you eat more. More calories, even when they're low fat, means you will gain more weight.

It's also important to remember that you need to have some fat in your diet for good health. Dietary fat is needed to carry vitamins A and E into your body, for example. You also need it for many other normal body functions.

Body fat isn't the same as dietary fat. Simply eating a diet relatively high in fat won't necessarily make you gain weight; likewise, eating a low-fat diet doesn't guarantee weight loss. In fact, there's no solid evidence linking a high-fat diet with obesity or a low-fat diet with thinness. Many people gain weight as they get older, for example, even as their intake of dietary fat remains the same. In the 1950s, most Americans got about 40 percent of their calories from fat. Today we get about 34 percent of our calories from fat on average, but we're fatter than ever—as mentioned, half of all American adults are now overweight.

And contrary to popular wisdom, it is possible to be too thin. Your body's fat deposits are used not only as a nutritional storehouse but also to cushion your organs and keep you warm, among other functions. If your fat deposits drop below normal levels, it can cause serious health problems, such as irregular menstruation and infertility in women.

RANKING THE FATS

Here's how the fats rank in terms of your health:

• **Polyunsaturated fats.** Not only good but essential. The omega-3 and omega-6 fatty acids are essential, meaning you need them to live and have to get them from your diet. However, not all polyunsaturated oils are equal, and getting the right balance of omega-3s and omega-6s is crucial to good health.

• **Monounsaturated fat.** Excellent. The best-known monounsaturated fat is olive oil, which has been shown to have a number of beneficial effects on health.

• **Saturated fat.** Bad—or at least not as good as monounsaturated or polyunsaturated fat. A substantial body of medical research suggests—but doesn't prove—that a diet high in saturated fats may lead to high blood cholesterol, which in turn leads to an increased risk of heart disease. On the other hand, the link between saturated fat and heart disease isn't really as strong as many people think it is. The same is true for the link between a high-fat diet and some types of cancer, such as colon cancer, breast cancer, prostate cancer, and endometrial cancer. The evidence so far is suggestive but far from conclusive.

• **Trans fat.** Deadly. These fats raise your blood cholesterol—and the more of them you eat, the higher your cholesterol will go. Avoid them.

• **Cholesterol.** Not good, but perhaps not as bad as you think. Like saturated fats, diets high in cholesterol are associated with high blood cholesterol and an increased risk of heart disease and stroke. Eating less cholesterol doesn't generally do much to lower your blood cholesterol, however. There's also some solid evidence that diets too low in cholesterol can lead to a greater chance of stroke and possibly cancer.

HOW MUCH FAT SHOULD YOU EAT?

The dietary guidelines for Americans put out by the United States Department of Agriculture (USDA), the Food and Drug Administration (FDA, which is part of the Department of Health and Human Services), and the National Cholesterol Education Program (NCEP) from the National Institutes of Health all strongly recommend that you get no more than 30 percent of your daily calories from fat. Of those 30 percent, they further recommend that only 10 percent come from saturated fats. The guidelines also recommend that you take in no more than 300 milligrams a day of cholesterol.

Many other medical organizations strongly endorse the basic 30 percent rule. The American Heart Association gets a little more detailed in its dietary guidelines for healthy American adults:

• Total fat intake should be no more than 30 percent of total calories.

• Saturated fat intake should be 8 to 10 percent of total calories.

• Polyunsaturated fat intake should be up to 10 percent of total calories.

• Monounsaturated fat intake should make up 15 percent of total calories.

• Cholesterol intake should be 300 milligrams or less per day.

Remember that the basic 30 percent–of–calories guideline applies to your average overall food intake over the course of a week or so. It doesn't apply to individual foods. In other words, it's perfectly okay to eat a normal portion of a food such as salmon, which gets 36 percent of its calories from fat, or nuts, which get anywhere from 75 to 90 percent of their calories from fat. The goal you're aiming for is an average of 30 percent of your total calories from fat from the total amount of the food you eat.

In practical terms, what does that work out to? Take a look at Table 1.1 to find out how many grams of fat and saturated fat are right for your average daily calorie level. When looking at this table, bear in mind that the average moderately active adult needs about 2,000 calories a day. If you're a lot more active, you need more calories; if you're inactive, you need fewer.

Table 1.1 Recommended Daily Amounts of Fat and Saturated Fat

Calorie Level	Total Fat (grams)	Saturated Fat (grams)
1,200	40 or less	11 to 13
1,500	50 or less	13 to 17
1,800	60 or less	16 to 20
2,000	67 or less	18 to 22
2,200	73 or less	20 to 24
2,500	83 or less	22 to 28
3,000	100 or less	27 to 33

Source: National Cholesterol Education Program

Table 1.2 presents another way to look at the right amount of fat for you, based on your body weight (assuming you're not overweight).

Table 1.2 Recommended Amounts of Daily Fat by Body Weight

Body Weight (pounds)	Total Fat (grams)
100 to 115	50
120 to 138	60
140 to 162	70
160 to 185	80

Source: National Cholesterol Education Program

If you're overweight or need to limit your fat intake because you have high cholesterol or another medical concern, you might need to limit your fat intake to 25 percent of your daily calories or even less.

As mentioned, there is a problem with lowering your fat intake too much. A 1998 study by the Department of Agriculture showed that more than half of the women who reduce their fat intake to less than 30 percent of their daily calories don't get the recommended daily intake of vitamins A and E, folic acid, calcium, iron, and zinc. If you take in under 2,000 calories a day, and if 30 percent or fewer of those calories are from fat, you might be shortchanging yourself on your overall nutrition. If you're cutting calories and fat because you're dieting, be sure you do it in a way that gives you all the essential nutrients. If you normally take in less than 2,000 calories a day (because you have a petite build, for instance), you still need to be sure you're getting enough vitamins from your diet and from supplements if necessary.

So far, no medical or government body has come out with a specific recommendation for how much trans fat you should eat. There's an easy rule of thumb to follow, however: as little as possible, and certainly no more than 5 grams a day.

TRACKING YOUR FAT

How can you know if your diet matches the guidelines for fat? It's fairly easy to keep track of your intake of total fat, saturated fat, and cholesterol, because this information is found on the food facts label for packaged foods. For meals out and unlabeled foods, you can check any of the many fat-counter books. Unfortunately, until the labeling requirement for trans fats goes into effect, you'd be in the dark about the levels of these dangerous fats in processed foods. You can make an educated guess, however, by using the information in Chapter 5 and the "Trans Fat Content of Selected Foods" table at the back of this book. And you can use the information in Chapter 6 on the food label to estimate your fat intake.

FAT AND THE FOOD PYRAMID

To make the dietary guidelines for Americans easier to understand, the well-known food pyramid was introduced in 1992. At the base of the pyramid are six to eleven servings daily of grains: bread, cereal, rice, and pasta. Higher up are three to five servings daily from the vegetable group, and two to four servings from the fruit group. Above that are two to three servings daily from the meat, poultry, fish, beans, eggs, and nuts group and two to three servings daily from the dairy foods group. At the very tip of the pyramid are fats, oils, and sweets, with the advice to use them sparingly. This advice corresponds to the dietary guideline to get less than 30 percent of your daily calories from fat.

The dietary guidelines for Americans and the food pyramid are now very widely accepted. The overall advice is sound, but looking at the food pyramid makes a major flaw in the dietary guidelines very apparent. Combining meat, fish, poultry, eggs, beans, and nuts into one food group ignores the differing fat contents of these foods. Red meat, poultry, and eggs contain saturated fat and cholesterol, so the suggestion to limit these to a maximum of three servings a day makes some sense. Fish contains little or no cholesterol, however, but it does contain highly beneficial omega-3 oils that can help prevent heart disease. Nuts contain no cholesterol at all, but they are rich in beneficial oils.

Two recent studies by researchers at Harvard Medical School have looked carefully at how adhering to the dietary guidelines for Americans translates into better health. Their conclusions? For both men and women, following the guidelines made virtually no difference at all in their risk of developing a major health problem such as stroke, heart disease, or cancer.[1]

Why aren't the dietary guidelines working as well as they should be? There are several possible reasons, according to the researchers. When a person's total fat intake is under 30 percent of calories, the diet may not contain enough beneficial unsaturated fats. Also, the carbohydrate base of the pyramid encourages people to eat more refined grains—and most processed baked goods are high not just in calories but in trans fats. And by combining red meat, fish, and nuts all in the same category, the guidelines actually discourage consumption of some healthy fats.

Does this mean that the dietary guidelines for fat should be ignored? No—but it does mean that you need to understand more about the fats in your diet to be sure you're getting the good ones and avoiding the bad ones. That's what the rest of this book explains.

Chapter Two

THE BAD FATS

Saturated fat and cholesterol fall into the "bad" fats category, but that description is actually a little harsh. Saturated fat in moderation is perfectly healthy, as is cholesterol. In fact, cholesterol is extremely important for your overall health. These fats become bad only when you eat too much of them, especially if you eat them as part of an overall diet that's high in trans fats and low in good fats.

SATURATED FAT IN YOUR DIET

Saturated fats are "hard" fats—they're generally solid or semisolid at room temperature. Good examples are butter, tallow (beef fat), and lard. Some tropical oils, such as coconut oil, are liquid at room temperature but still very high in saturated fat.

All fats, however, are really mixtures of saturated and unsaturated fatty acids. Animal fats, such as lard and butter, are high in saturated fat, but they also contain high amounts of monounsaturated fat. In fact, lard has more monounsaturated fat than saturated fat per serving. Like all animal fats, lard contains some cholesterol (12 milligrams per 1-tablespoon serving), but it has far more monounsaturated fat than the supposedly more healthful vegetable oils such as soybean or corn.

Meat, poultry, eggs, fish, shellfish, and whole-milk dairy

products, such as cheese and butter, contain saturated fat and cholesterol. Dishes made using these basic ingredients will contain saturated fat and cholesterol as well. Fruits, vegetables, and grains have no or very little saturated fat; nuts have some, but not a lot, and plenty of good fats that more than compensate.

Although animal foods such as beef usually are considered as sources of only saturated fat, the fat in these foods is also a mixture of saturated, monounsaturated, and polyunsaturated fat. A 3.5-ounce broiled hamburger, for instance, contains 19.7 grams of fat. Of that, 7.7 grams is saturated fat, but 8.6 grams is monounsaturated fat. Likewise, a 3.5-ounce pork chop has 22.1 grams of fat. Of that, 8.0 grams is saturated fat and 10.2 grams is monounsaturated fat.

Sometimes tropical oils, such as palm oil, coconut oil, and palm kernel oil, are used in cookies, crackers, other baked goods, and nondairy creamers, often in place of partially hydrogenated vegetable oil (trans fat). Because these tropical oils are highly saturated, consumer outcry has led many food manufacturers to remove them and replace them with trans fat. But substituting trans fats for tropical oils isn't really more healthful at all—in fact, it's worse.

What makes saturated fat so bad for you? That's a good question—and one that doesn't have a clear answer yet. In general, however, research that looks at large groups of people has consistently shown that overall, the people who eat the most fat of all kinds also tend to have the most heart disease. The research behind the recommendations to cut dietary fat is not without controversy, however. Some of the original studies, such as the famous Seven Countries study done in the 1950s, didn't take into account cigarette smoking and other risk factors and also looked very selectively at some of the data. Other studies since then have shown that people who eat a lot of saturated fat don't eat much in the way of fresh fruits and vegetables and unsaturated oils. Many researchers believe that this lack, not the amount of saturated fat in the diet, is the real cause of heart disease. Extensive health data gathered by food consumption studies run by the Harvard School of Public Health have all shown that total fat consumption has little or no relation to your risk of heart disease.

What about stroke? Here, too, the assumption that having a high intake of saturated fat increases your risk of stroke has been shown to be false. In fact, eating too little saturated fat actually may increase your risk of stroke. The male participants in the well-known Framingham Heart Study who were most likely to have a stroke were the ones who ate the least fat overall and also ate the least saturated and monounsaturated fats. The men least likely to have a stroke? The ones who had the highest fat intake.[1]

THE CHOLESTEROL IN YOUR BODY

After saturated fat, cholesterol is the fat doctors warn most against (even though cholesterol isn't really a fat). That's because elevated levels of total blood cholesterol are closely associated with heart disease and stroke. Also, recent research suggests that the combination of high cholesterol and high blood pressure in middle age makes a person much more likely to get Alzheimer's disease later in life.[2]

Eating a lot of high-cholesterol foods may play a role in raising your blood cholesterol, and eating a low-fat, low-cholesterol diet may play a role in lowering it. But despite everything you've read about the dangers of high blood cholesterol, low cholesterol isn't always healthier. In fact, low levels of cholesterol (below 160 milligrams per deciliter [mg/dL]) are associated with a higher risk of premature death from stroke, respiratory illness, and cancer. Low cholesterol also may play a role in depression and some cognitive problems in elderly people.

To avoid some of the confusion that surrounds the whole question of fat in the diet, it's important to distinguish between the cholesterol in your diet and the cholesterol in your body. Let's start by taking a closer look at what cholesterol really is.

As explained in Chapter 1, cholesterol is a lipid, or fatlike substance, but it's not technically a fat—it's sort of a cousin to fat. An important difference between cholesterol and fat is that your body doesn't burn cholesterol for energy, so cholesterol has no calories. Your body does use cholesterol for other important purposes, however. In fact, cholesterol is essential for your health—you *have* to have it. Most of the cholesterol you need is manufactured in your body; you need only small amounts from food.

In total, you have about 150 grams, or about 5 ounces, of cholesterol in your body. Most of it is in your cell membranes; only about 7 grams of cholesterol circulates in your bloodstream.

What does your body do with all that cholesterol? A lot of very important things that you literally can't live without. Cholesterol is a major component of the membranes that support every cell in your body. Because the cell membrane regulates what goes into and out of the cell, it's crucial that it be strong yet flexible. Cholesterol is what gives the cell membrane its integrity.

You also need cholesterol to make steroid hormones, such as estrogen, progesterone, and testosterone, as well as adrenal hormones, such as aldosterone, which regulates the amount of water in your body, and cortisone, which regulates many functions, including inflammation. Hormones keep your body's normal functions in balance—and without cholesterol, your body can't make them.

You need cholesterol to manufacture vitamin D in your body; this process in turn is crucial for regulating the amounts of calcium and phosphorus in your blood and in your bones.

Bile acids, which are crucial for the proper digestion of fats and oils in the diet, are made from cholesterol.

WHERE CHOLESTEROL COMES FROM

The cholesterol in your body comes from two sources: your-self and the foods you eat. Most cells in your body can make small amounts of cholesterol in order to maintain their membranes. In addition, your liver, intestines, adrenal glands, and sex glands make cholesterol.

Your body makes cholesterol as it needs it, mostly in your liver, at the rate of about 800 to 1,500 milligrams a day. The average American also eats about 300 to 450 milligrams or more cholesterol daily, but of that amount, not more than half—and perhaps only as little as 10 percent—is actually absorbed into the body.

In general, if you eat more cholesterol, your body com-pensates by making less, and vice versa. The compensation depends on complex feedback loops that signal your cells and organs to change their level of cholesterol production, but in some people, the control system doesn't work very well. They could end up with high levels of cholesterol in their blood, as is discussed a little later in this chapter.

Once your body manufactures cholesterol, it can't break it down again. The only way to remove it from your blood-stream is through the bile acids, which are produced in your liver and used as part of the digestive process. Some of the cholesterol in them is reabsorbed through your intestines, but most of the bile acids and the cholesterol they carry are excreted.

THE CHOLESTEROL IN YOUR BLOOD

High levels of cholesterol in your blood are believed to be the major cause of atheromas—soft, fatty deposits and streaks on the linings of your arteries, especially the arteries that nourish your heart, brain, and kidneys. Atheromas even-tually harden to form arterial plaque—stiff, fatty deposits that clog the arteries. A plaque deposit narrows the artery and keeps blood from flowing through it easily. When that happens, the backed-up blood may form a clot that blocks the artery, or a piece of the plaque may break off and block the artery. In either case, the result can be deadly: a heart attack if the artery feeds the heart, a stroke if it's in the brain.

GOOD AND BAD CHOLESTEROL

Cholesterol is transported through your body in the form of lipoproteins—complexes of cholesterol and protein. There are several kinds of lipoproteins, but the two most important are low-density lipoprotein, or LDL cholesterol, and high-density lipoprotein, or HDL cholesterol. LDL cholesterol carries fat and cholesterol from your liver, where the cholesterol is manufactured, to the parts of your body that need it. HDL cholesterol carries unused cholesterol back to your liver, where it is recycled into bile acids.

In general, LDL cholesterol is considered the "bad" cholesterol, because high levels of LDL in your blood are associated with a greater risk of heart disease and stroke from clogged arteries. Although researchers still aren't quite sure about how the process works, most believe that LDL cholesterol oxidizes easily—in effect, it turns rancid. In a complex process that isn't fully understood, oxidized LDL cholesterol seems to become "sticky" and more likely to form fatty deposits.

Offsetting the LDL cholesterol, however, is HDL cholesterol, the "good" cholesterol. HDL clears cholesterol from your bloodstream and carries it back to your liver. The higher your HDL level, the more cholesterol is being removed from your bloodstream before it has a chance to oxidize.

For a long time, doctors thought that the total amount of cholesterol in your blood was all they needed to look at.

More recently, they've realized that the proportions of LDL and HDL are much more important. Ideally, you want to have a relatively low amount of LDL cholesterol and a relatively high amount of HDL cholesterol in your blood.

Doctors also have recently realized that there is more to your blood lipid profile than just cholesterol. The current guidelines from the National Cholesterol Education Program (NCEP) now recommend checking your level of triglycerides (TG), another fatty substance in the blood. That's because the combination of high LDL, low HDL, and high TG is especially deadly—if you have it, the chances are good there's a heart attack in your future.

THE LATEST CHOLESTEROL GUIDELINES

Every few years, the NCEP convenes a group of experts to look at the cholesterol guidelines and make recommendations. The third Adult Treatment Panel (ATP III) of twenty-seven leading experts issued the latest NCEP guidelines for healthy blood lipid levels in May 2001. Here's what they call for:

- Total cholesterol of 200 mg/dL or less.

- LDL cholesterol of 100 mg/dL or less.

- HDL cholesterol of 40 mg/dL or more. HDL of 60 mg/dL or more is considered protective against heart disease.

- TG of 40 mg/dL or more.

The NCEP didn't specify new levels for high triglycerides, primarily because a low-fat diet and cholesterol-lowering drugs have little effect on this number. Losing weight, getting more exercise, and reducing your cholesterol numbers seem to be the only way to get your TG level down. In fact, in some cases a low-fat diet actually can raise TG levels while lowering HDL levels—exactly the opposite of what you want.

In general, a TG level of 150 mg/dL or more is considered high. The lower your TG, the better. Ideally, your HDL and TG levels should be in a one-to-one ratio or close to it.

The new guidelines are a lot more aggressive than the previous guidelines. They call for a major focus on identifying people who have multiple risk factors for coronary heart disease, such as high cholesterol and high blood pressure. They also call for new dietary and lifestyle recommendations and for more use of cholesterol-lowering drugs to reduce cholesterol levels when dietary changes don't help enough. The panel estimated that some 65 million American adults need to be on dietary treatment for high cholesterol, up from 52 million, and about 36 million need prescription cholesterol-lowering drugs, up from 13 million.

NEW DIETARY GUIDELINES

The current dietary guidelines for healthy adults with normal cholesterol levels are very familiar by now: Get no more than 30 percent of your calories from fat, including no more than 10 percent of those calories from saturated fat, and limit your dietary cholesterol intake to 300 mg a day.

The new NCEP dietary guidelines for people at risk of heart disease reduce the fat and cholesterol in the diet even more—and because according to the new standards a lot more adults are at risk, the new guidelines soon may become the standard for all adults.

The new NCEP guidelines recommend both dietary and lifestyle changes as the first line of attack against high cholesterol. Instead of the old Step I and Step II diets, which called for less dietary fat, the new guidelines call for TLC—therapeutic lifestyle changes. The TLC approach combines dietary and lifestyle components:

• Limit total fat intake to 35 percent of daily calories, but only if most of it comes from unsaturated fats.

• Reduce saturated fat intake to less than 7 percent of daily calories.

• Reduce cholesterol intake to less than 200 mg a day.

• Use 2 grams a day of margarines and salad dressings containing plant stanols and sterols.

• Eat foods high in soluble fiber such as whole grains, beans, peas, and fruits and vegetables. The goal is 10 to 25 grams of fiber daily. A diet high in soluble fiber helps reduce cholesterol levels.

• Lose weight. LDL cholesterol goes down when you lose weight—even if you lose it by liposuction!

• Increase physical activity. LDL cholesterol goes down, HDL cholesterol goes up, and triglycerides go down when you exercise, even if you don't change your diet. But if you go on the NCEP diet and also exercise, your blood lipids will probably improve even more.[3]

One big problem with the new dietary guidelines is that they don't specifically warn against trans fats, even though these fats are twice as deadly as saturated fat. This is all the more surprising when you look at the summary of the scientific conference that announced the new guidelines. In its conclusions, the researchers state: "Based on a large body of evidence, it is apparent that the optimal diet for reducing risk of chronic diseases is one in which saturated fatty acids are reduced and trans fatty acids from manufactured fats are virtually eliminated."[4] Eliminating this deadly fat from the diet gets rid of a major source of artery-clogging blood lipids.

What can you do to cut saturated fat and cholesterol from your diet? A lot—and as you'll discover later in this book, it's easier than you think.

Chapter Three
THE KILLER FAT

Of all the fats you can eat, trans fats, also known as trans fatty acids or partially hydrogenated vegetable oils, are the worst—no question. In fact, today there's a very solid body of scientific evidence showing that these artificially created fats are twice as dangerous to your heart health as saturated fats.

What makes trans fats so deadly? Gram for gram, trans fats are twice as bad for you as saturated fat. That means each gram of trans fat you eat is twice as likely to end up clogging your arteries and causing heart disease or a stroke.

Trans fats start out as inexpensive monounsaturated or polyunsaturated vegetable oils, such as corn oil, soybean oil, or canola oil. To turn natural vegetable oils into trans fats, the oils first are chemically stripped of their linolenic acid, which immediately lowers their health value. The remaining oil is then processed using heat and a metal catalyst (a substance that speeds up a chemical reaction), such as nickel, to force hydrogen atoms back into them—that's why trans fats are also called partially hydrogenated vegetable oils. In effect, the processing makes the oils more saturated. The longer the hydrogenation process is allowed to continue, the more saturated the vegetable oil becomes.

The hydrogenation process forces the fat molecules in the vegetable oil to change their shapes from their normal slightly curved, C shape into long strands.

Why go through all this processing? Because by altering

the shape and chemical structure of the vegetable oil molecules, hydrogenation changes slippery liquid oils into thicker, more viscous liquids or semisolids that hold their shape at room temperature. The more hydrogenated the fat is, the harder it gets and the better it keeps—partially hydrogenated vegetable oils don't turn rancid.

To food manufacturers, trans fats are wonderful. They're very inexpensive, they're flavorless, and they don't go bad. That means trans fats can give foods such as cookies the same satisfying "mouth feel" that comes from more expensive fats such as butter, but for much less money—and the products last much longer on the shelf.

Trans fats are ideal for high-profit baked goods like cakes, crackers, muffins, pies, and sugary snack foods. Check the label on almost any cookie or snack cake package and you'll see that partially hydrogenated vegetable oil is the third ingredient, right after the enriched white flour and sugar. It's the trans fat that makes the pie crusts flaky, the cookies "buttery," and the frostings firm.

Fast-food restaurants and snack-food manufacturers love trans fats for two very good reasons: They can withstand high temperatures without breaking down or smoking, and they make fried foods nicely crisp. That makes lightly hydrogenated vegetable oil ideal for deep-frying french fries and other fast foods, for making high-profit convenience foods such as fried chicken and fish sticks, and for making salty snack foods such as potato chips and corn chips.

The oil industry loves trans fats because it can turn its low-profit liquid vegetable oils into high-profit margarines. Consumers buy margarine because it is less expensive than butter—and because for years they were falsely told that margarine is healthier for the heart than butter.

WHAT'S WRONG WITH TRANS FATS

If partially hydrogenated vegetable oils were called what they truly are, partially saturated vegetable oils, it would be much easier to understand why they're so bad for you. Trans fats are more saturated than natural vegetable oil, although they are less saturated than animal fat or butter. A diet high in saturated fats of any kind is likely to raise your blood cholesterol level and cause heart disease. For that reason alone, then, you can see that trans fats wouldn't be all that good for you, although they arguably are better than an equal amount of a more saturated fat such as lard.

What makes trans fats so very dangerous, however, is that they actually are even *worse* for your heart than saturated fats. Scientific evidence shows that trans fats raise your total blood cholesterol even *more* than saturated fats. Even worse, trans fats don't just raise your LDL ("bad") cholesterol, they *lower* your HDL ("good") cholesterol. In fact, the combined bad effect of trans fatty acids on your LDL/HDL ratio is *twice* that of saturated fats.[1] Even worse than that, trans fats *raise* the level of triglycerides (TG) in your blood.[2] Recent research has shown that the combination of low HDL and high TG raises your risk of heart disease sharply. In fact, low HDL/high TG is probably the most accurate predictor that a heart attack is in your future.[3] A number of studies also have shown that trans fats raise the level of a type of fat known as lipoprotein(a) in your blood.[4] Although researchers still aren't certain why lipoprotein(a) is bad, they do know that the more you have, the more likely you are to have heart disease.

Not only do trans fats lower your HDL cholesterol and raise your LDL cholesterol, they also make your blood vessels less flexible. When a group of healthy, nonsmoking volunteers ate a diet high in trans fat for four weeks, the ability of their blood vessels to open wider in response to increased blood flow was reduced by 29 percent. Because reduced blood vessel function is a clear marker of increased risk of heart disease, this is yet more evidence of how harmful trans fats can be.[5]

Ever since the 1960s, when trans fats became very common in the American diet, researchers have suspected that they were at least one of the culprits in the rising tide of heart disease. The real proof didn't start to come in until the 1980s, and starting in the 1990s, the scientific evidence against trans fats has become much, much stronger.

Two important studies in 1994 by Walter C. Willett and Alberto Ascherio, leading epidemiologists from the Harvard School of Public Health, showed that overall, the people who eat the most trans fats are also the most likely to develop heart disease. Specifically, their studies showed a strong and significant positive association between trans fat intake and the risk of having a heart attack.[6] According to these experts, about 30,000 premature coronary heart disease deaths annually—and possibly as many as 100,000 deaths—can be blamed on consumption of trans fats.[7]

Two important epidemiological studies have looked at the relationship between the amount of trans fats in the diets of large groups of people and their rates of heart disease over the long run. Both studies showed that trans fatty acids had an adverse effect: The relative risk of coronary heart disease increased as consumption of trans fats went up. In other words, just as the earlier Harvard study showed, the people who ate the most trans fats had a markedly higher risk of heart disease when compared to similar people who ate the least trans fats. And in both studies, the relative risks of heart disease from trans fats were *higher* than the risks from saturated fats. In the Health Professionals Follow-Up Study, an increase of just 2 percent in a man's intake of trans fats increased his relative risk of heart disease by about 35 percent.[8] In the Nurses' Health Study, women who increased their intake of trans fats by only 2 to 3 grams a days increased their risk of coronary artery disease by 21 percent. Women who replaced 5 percent of their calories from saturated fat with unsaturated fat had a 42 percent decrease in their risk of coronary artery disease. Women who replaced just 2 percent of their calories from trans fats with unsaturated fat, however, saw their risk decrease 53 percent.

In other words, cutting your trans fats intake by only 2 percent reduces your risk of heart disease by more than half—even more than cutting your saturated fat intake by 5 percent.[9]

Based on the mounting evidence, in 1997 the American Heart Association (AHA) issued a medical/scientific statement on trans fats and their relation to blood lipid levels and the risk of developing cardiovascular disease. The AHA believes "it is prudent to recommend that naturally occurring unhydrogenated oil be used when possible and attempts made to substitute unhydrogenated oil for hydrogenated or saturated fat in processed foods. Additionally, the recommendation to substitute softer for harder margarines and cooking fats seems justified."[10] In 1999 a major article in the prestigious *New England Journal of Medicine* by three leading researchers reviewed all the research on trans fats and made a powerful case against them.[11] Here's their conclusion: "Metabolic and epidemiologic studies indicate an adverse effect of trans fatty acids on the risk of coronary heart disease. Furthermore, on a per-gram basis, the adverse effect of trans fatty acids appears to be stronger than that of saturated fatty acids." The authors go on to make a very strong argument for insisting that the amount of trans fats in a product be included on the food label.

Trans fats are more saturated than unprocessed vegetable oils, but they're less saturated than animal fats—and they don't have any cholesterol. What makes them raise your blood lipids so much? Researchers still aren't sure, but the current thinking is that these fats are so unnatural that your body isn't designed to deal with them. Like other fats you eat, some molecules of trans fats end up in your cell membranes. There they play a role in how the membrane allows nutrients to enter the cell. Recent test-tube research suggests that when trans fatty acids are incorporated into the membranes of the cells that line the coronary arteries, the cells allow more calcium to enter them—especially if the cells are also low in magnesium. Because the first step toward narrowed and clogged arteries from atherosclerosis is calcium in those artery cells, and because many Americans in fact do eat a diet low in magnesium (because we don't eat enough fresh fruits, vegetables, and nuts), this research may be an important clue about how trans fats do their damage.[12] Other researchers believe that trans fats in the cell membrane also interfere with other normal cell functions. Trans fats may affect the body's use of essential fatty acids by interfering with or blocking some crucial pathways, such as hormone production.

Pretty convincing, isn't it? The FDA thinks so, too. The FDA is working on labeling regulations that will force food manufacturers to list the trans fat content of a food on the label. Until the new regulations go into effect, however, you're on your own when it comes to finding—and avoiding—the trans fats in foods. To learn where the trans fats are in the foods you eat, see the fat counter at the back of the book for a breakdown for many common foods.

TRANS FATS AND DIABETES

The obesity epidemic of the twenty-first century has spawned another epidemic: diabetes. The number of people in the United States with type 2 (adult-onset) diabetes is now nearly 16 million, or about 6 percent of the population—and it is rising fast, with about 800,000 new cases diagnosed each year. The annual direct medical costs of diabetes-related illnesses are estimated at $44 billion—and rising fast, as well.

The risk of developing type 2 diabetes goes up sharply the more you weigh and the older you get. The more overweight you are, the more likely you are to develop diabetes by middle age. With diabetes comes a long list of serious health consequences, particularly a sharply increased risk of heart disease and other problems caused by clogged arteries. In fact, the risk of heart disease is so great in type 2 diabetics that it is now standard practice for doctors to treat these patients as heart patients and prescribe cholesterol-lowering drugs, even if they don't show signs of heart disease yet.

If clogged arteries are a major health consequence of diabetes, you might think that eating a high-fat diet would play a role in increasing your risk of developing diabetes. In fact, dietary fat does indeed play a very important role in diabetes. Recent research strongly suggests that of all the dietary fats, trans fats are the ones most closely related to developing diabetes.

In a major study published in 2001, researchers from the Harvard School of Public Health used data from the Nurses' Health Study of some 84,000 women over fourteen years to compare dietary fat intake and the risk of developing diabetes. The results were very revealing. Total fat intake had little effect on which women in the group developed diabetes. In other words, the women who ate the most fats overall had very little greater risk of diabetes than the women who ate the least. Similarly, the women who ate the most saturated fats or monounsaturated fats had very little greater risk of diabetes than those who ate the least.

The women who ate the most polyunsaturated fats, however, had a sharply *decreased* risk of diabetes compared to those who ate the least. All it took to reduce their risk of diabetes by 37 percent was getting 5 percent more of their daily calories from polyunsaturated fats.

The most shocking revelation of the study, however, was the impact of trans fats. The women who ate the most trans fats had a sharply *increased* risk of diabetes compared to those who ate the least. The effect was dramatic. An increase of just 2 percent in their daily calories from trans fats raised their risk of diabetes by 39 percent.[13] Overall, if everyone at risk of diabetes replaced just 2 percent of daily calories from trans fats with polyunsaturates, the overall incidence of diabetes would drop by a massive 40 percent.[14]

Trans fats alone can't be blamed for type 2 diabetes, of course. Obesity, inactivity, a diet high in refined carbohydrates, and many other factors all play a role as well. But a diet high in trans fats goes hand-in-hand with an obesity-causing diet high in refined carbohydrates. By eliminating the trans fats, you also eliminate some other contributing factors to diabetes. And by substituting polyunsaturated fats for trans fats—by eating more fish and less cake, for example—your risk of diabetes is driven down even further.

TRANS FATS AND CANCER

There's no arguing with the evidence linking trans fats and heart disease, but the link with cancer is less clear. Even so, recent research has pointed to a possible role for trans fats in causing cancer.

The ongoing EURAMIC study has been looking at the connection among antioxidants, heart attacks, and breast cancer in European women for a number of years. In 1997, researchers reported that women diagnosed with breast cancer had higher levels of trans fatty acids in their body fat than healthy women. The women with the highest trans fat levels had a 40 percent greater risk of breast cancer.[15] The study looked only at 698 postmenopausal women, however, and it's far from conclusive—more research with larger numbers of women is definitely needed.[16] And despite years of research, there's still no conclusive evidence that a high-fat diet in general increases the risk of breast cancer; likewise, there's no conclusive evidence that a low-fat diet decreases the risk.[17]

What about other cancers and trans fats? There may be a link with colon cancer. In a 2000 study, researchers compared a group of patients found to have colorectal adenomas with a healthy group. The cancer patients were more likely to eat a diet high in sweetened baked goods and oils and condiments than the healthy people.[18] Here, too, however, the number of people studied was small (only about 650) and the results weren't all that strong.

So far, no good study has shown for sure that trans fats cause cancer. The evidence doesn't rule trans fats out, however, and it does suggest possible links. Cutting trans fats from your diet certainly won't increase your risk of cancer, however, and it may well reduce it.

TRANS FATS AND ASTHMA

In recent years, there has been a huge increase in the number of children with asthma in the industrialized world. A lot of factors have been blamed, including increased air pollution, but it's possible that diet plays an important role. Children who eat the most fresh fruits and vegetables are the least likely to develop asthma; normal-weight children are less likely to develop asthma than overweight children. Fatty acids in the diet also may play a role. Recent research in Finland suggests that the children who eat the most margarine and the least butter are also the most likely to develop asthma due to allergies. In the study, the children with allergic asthma ate about 8 grams of margarine for every 1,000 calories; children without allergies ate only 6 grams per 1,000 calories.[19] Another study in Australia has shown that toddlers who eat large amounts of margarine and foods fried in vegetable oil may be twice as likely to develop asthma as similar kids who eat less of these foods.[20] This research is too preliminary to be anything more than suggestive, but it does point in an interesting direction.

TRANS FATS AND YOUR EYESIGHT

The leading cause of blindess and vision impairment for people over age fifty-five is age-related macular degeneration (AMD). For a long time the only known risk factor for this incurable disease was smoking, but recent research has shown that eating a lot of snack foods, which are high in trans fats, is a risk factor, as well. In fact, if you eat a lot of trans fats from snack foods like chips and candy, your risk of AMD is roughly twice that of someone who eats only small amounts of trans fats.[21]

As research into trans fats continues, the dangers these artificial fats pose will almost certainly become even more obvious. Why wait for more evidence? The time to reduce the amount of trans fats in your diet is now.

Chapter Four

TRIMMING THE FAT, CUTTING THE CHOLESTEROL

You want to trim the fat from your diet, but where do you begin? The typical American diet makes it very easy to eat way too much saturated fat, trans fats, and cholesterol and very hard to get plenty of whole grains, fruits, and vegetables. A typical fast-food meal of a quarter-pound hamburger with cheese, a large order of fries, and a chocolate milkshake contains a whopping 40.5 grams of fat—of which 23.5 grams, or more than half, are saturated. That doesn't include the 15 grams of trans fat found in the fries. This typical meal also contains 135 mg cholesterol and 1,400 calories. If you choose the chicken nuggets instead of the hamburger, you won't be saving all that much in fat. A nine-piece serving of chicken nuggets has 25 grams of fat, including 5 grams from saturated fat and about 20 grams from trans fat, and 80 mg of cholesterol. It has 430 calories, identical to the quarter-pound hamburger without the cheese.

To trim the saturated fat in your diet, some of those high-fat fast-food meals will have to go. This is harder than you might think, because the average American eats in a fast-food restaurant of some sort at least twice a week. The whole point of fast food, of course, is those delicious burgers, fries, and shakes, so it will take real dedication to go for a grilled chicken salad, baked potato, and diet soft drink instead. There's nothing wrong with an occasional meal from the drive-through window, but realistically speaking, the best way to avoid fast-food fat is to avoid those restaurants as much as possible.

In general, you can reduce your saturated fat intake by eating meats that have been broiled or baked. Choose lean cuts of meat and remove the skin from chicken. Unfortunately, there's no way to reduce the cholesterol in animal foods. The only way to get less cholesterol is to simply eat less of these foods. In general, poultry and fish have less cholesterol than red meat, so substituting chicken for steak will reduce your cholesterol intake somewhat.

The American Heart Association suggests in general that you choose fish, shellfish, poultry without the skin, and trimmed lean meats. Your daily intake of these foods should be no more than 6 ounces, cooked. Another excellent way to cut saturated fat and cholesterol is to substitute dried beans, peas, lentils, or tofu (soybean curd) for meat. One cup of cooked beans, peas, or lentils, or 3 ounces of tofu, counts as a 3-ounce meat serving. (To help you visualize this, a 3-ounce serving of meat is about the size of a deck of cards. For poultry, half a chicken breast or chicken leg with thigh is about 3 ounces.)

To reduce the saturated fat and cholesterol content of meat, choose lean beef cuts: round, sirloin, chuck, and loin. Choose choice or select grades of beef; prime is higher in fat. Look for lean or extra-lean ground beef, with no more than 15 percent fat. And avoid organ meats such as liver, kidneys, and brains—they are very high in cholesterol.

How you cook affects the fat contents. Instead of frying, prepare meats by baking, broiling, roasting, or stir-frying. Pour off the extra fat.

EGGS OR NOT?

When it comes to high-cholesterol foods, eggs are high on the list. One large egg contains about 200 milligrams of cholesterol—or roughly two-thirds of your daily allowance if you need to follow the NCEP guidelines. Doctors often suggest cutting back on eggs as a good way to reduce your cholesterol intake. On the other hand, eggs have been shown to help raise HDL cholesterol, which offsets their high cholesterol content somewhat. Eggs are an excellent source of other nutrients, such as high-quality protein, vitamin E, folate and other B vitamins, and iron. Eggs also contain the nutrients lutein and zeaxanthin, which can help protect your eyesight. In addition, lutein has recently been shown to help prevent the narrowing and thickening of arteries that can lead to heart attack and stroke.[1] Eggs are also a good source of desirable omega-3 fatty acids.

A study in 1999 from the Harvard School of Public Health suggests that eating one egg a day is unlikely to have any substantial impact on your risk of coronary heart disease or stroke if you're basically healthy. If you're diabetic, however, eating eggs often could increase your risk of coronary heart disease.[2]

The cholesterol in eggs is all found in the yolks, so you might try omelets made with only egg whites. Most people don't find that very appealing, so they try the convenient (but pricey) egg substitutes found in the dairy case at the supermarket. Egg substitutes are made from modified egg whites. They're fat free and cholesterol free and have some added vitamins, but they're missing the important good fats and the zeaxanthin and lutein.

Overall, it's probably healthier—and certainly tastier—to eat whole eggs less often rather than egg whites or egg substitutes more often. If your cholesterol is normal, limit your egg consumption to an average of one egg a day. If you have high cholesterol or diabetes, discuss with your doctor whether you should limit eggs.

FIBER LOWERS CHOLESTEROL

Reducing your total dietary cholesterol is the first step toward lowering your blood cholesterol. The next dietary step is increasing the amount of fiber in your diet.

There are two kinds of dietary fiber: soluble and insoluble. Soluble fiber is basically the indigestible parts, mostly cell walls, of plant foods. When soluble fiber is combined with water, it forms a soft gel in your intestines. The gel bulks up the intestinal contents and keeps them moving smoothly through your system.

The other kind of fiber is insoluble fiber, which is basically cellulose, the main fiber in the cell walls of all plant foods. Insoluble fiber absorbs water but doesn't dissolve in it—bran, for example, is high in insoluble fiber. Insoluble fiber is excellent for adding bulk to your intestinal contents.

The best dietary sources of both kinds of fiber are fresh fruits and vegetables with their peels (apple peels are 15 percent soluble fiber), cooked dried beans, whole grains, nuts, and seeds. In general, the fiber in plant foods is about 35 percent insoluble fiber and 45 percent soluble fiber. (The rest is miscellaneous other types of fiber.)

Soluble fiber is particularly helpful for reducing your cholesterol level. That's because your liver uses some of the cholesterol in your body to make bile acids, which are excreted into your small intestine as a normal part of the digestive process. If you eat a diet high in soluble fiber, a lot of the cholesterol-containing bile acids are bound up in the fiber as it moves through you. The cholesterol ends up being eliminated from your body instead of being reabsorbed. This lowers your blood cholesterol levels, because your liver now has to pull cholesterol from your blood to make bile acids.

A number of studies since the early 1980s have shown that soluble fiber, especially oat bran, works to lower blood cholesterol.[3] The effect is small, but it's enough to be significant—regularly eating soluble fiber can lower your LDL cholesterol level by a few percentage points. In combination with other dietary steps, that adds up. And even a 1 percent reduction in your LDL cholesterol translates into a 2 percent reduction in your risk of heart disease.

Based on the oat bran studies, in 1997 the FDA gave the food industry permission to make health claims for soluble fiber on food labels. As long as the food contains at least 0.75 grams of soluble fiber per serving, the label can say "This food, as part of a diet low in saturated fat and cholesterol, may reduce the risk of heart disease." Because wheat bran and oat bran are good sources of soluble fiber, you'll see the claim on oatmeal containers, some cereal boxes, and some breads. Bear in mind, however, that it will take several months of diligent oatmeal eating before you'll see any improvement in your cholesterol level.

How much soluble fiber is enough? According to the new NCEP guidelines, 10 to 25 grams a day. The more the better, however, according to the American Heart Association, National Institutes of Health, and American Cancer Association. These organizations all recommend 20 to 30 grams of fiber—both insoluble and soluble—a day. The FDA has set the daily reference value for fiber at 25 grams. To put that in perspective, the average American eats only about 12 grams of fiber a day. That's nowhere near enough. Two important studies, both published in the prestigious *Journal of the American Medical Association,* have shown that a diet rich in dietary fiber plays a major role in reducing the risk of heart disease. The first study, published in 1996, looked at the diets of nearly 44,000 American men. The men who ate the most fiber had a 41 percent lower risk of coronary heart disease than those who ate the least fiber. The study also showed that adding fiber to the diet reduces the risk of heart disease. By adding 10 grams of fiber to their daily diet, the men in the study who ate the least fiber reduced their risk of heart disease by 19 percent.[4]

The second study looked at the diets of some 68,000 women. The women who ate the most fiber had a 23 percent lower risk of coronary heart disease than the women who ate the least fiber. The benefits of the fiber kicked in the most for the women whose intake was an average of 23 grams a day. The women in the low-fiber group ate only 11.5 grams of fiber a day—very close to the American average.[5] Evidence shows that 25 grams of fiber a day is good for your cholesterol level—the fiber lowers your LDL cholesterol by a few points, but you might still need drugs to get it down to safe levels.

What if you were to eat 100 grams of fiber a day? Research shows that such a high-fiber diet would *really* lower your LDL cholesterol. In a 2001 study comparing different levels of fiber in the diet, the subjects who ate a vegetarian diet containing 100 grams of fiber from leafy vegetables, fruits, nuts, and whole grains lowered their total cholesterol by about 20 percent and their LDL cholesterol by about 30 percent—equivalent to the effect of cholesterol-lowering statin drugs.[6] Of course, it's hard to stick to a diet so high in fiber, but the research seems to suggest the more fiber the better, especially when it's substituted for high-fat foods.

It's easy to add more fiber to your diet. The more processed a food is, the less fiber it's likely to contain, so substitute whole-wheat bread and pasta for the stuff made with highly processed white flour. Switch to a bran cereal or oatmeal for breakfast—and top it with some fresh fruit. Eat more salads and vegetables and fewer french fries, and have a piece of fresh fruit or a carrot or celery stalk instead of a cookie. For a more substantial snack, try a handful of nuts. All it takes is a few minor changes and you'll be eating more fiber—and incidentally getting better overall nutrition.

Adding too much fiber all at once, however, can cause unpleasant side effects such as gas and bloating. Add the fiber gradually and give your digestive system time to adjust.

CHOLESTEROL-LOWERING SPREADS

Sterols, the plant equivalent of cholesterol, are found naturally in vegetable fats and oils. Some vegetable oils, such as sesame oil and corn oil, are naturally high in plant sterols; so are sunflower seeds, rice bran, peanuts, and green peas.

One particular type of sterol, sitosterol, has been shown to have a cholesterol-lowering effect when it's eaten on a regular basis. In a hardened form, it can be made into a margarine and used as a spread or topping.

Sterol esters work because they confuse your body and interfere with the absorption of cholesterol in your intestines. A number of studies have shown that margarines made with sterol esters are helpful for lowering cholesterol.[7] A 1999 study showed that eating 2 grams a day of the margarine can lower LDL cholesterol an average of 8.1 percent. The margarine didn't raise HDL levels, however, and it had no effect on triglycerides. The evidence from this study and earlier ones was enough to convince the FDA. In 2000 the FDA allowed the manufacturers of Take Control® and Benecol® to state on the food labels that these products have been proven to lower cholesterol and may lower the risk of heart disease when part of a diet low in saturated fat and cholesterol.

The research suggests that 3.4 grams of plant stanol esters daily is the amount needed to lower LDL cholesterol levels. Each one-tablespoon serving of Benecol contains 1.7 grams of plant stanol esters, so you'd have to eat two servings daily to get the benefit. It's not clear if eating more will help more, although it won't hurt.

There are some drawbacks to the sterol margarines. They're very pricey, costing about 25 cents a serving. A 1-tablespoon serving has 50 calories, which means that 3 tablespoons a day adds up to 150 calories—about 7 percent of a 2,000-calorie diet. Sterol margarines may turn out to be one of the easiest ways to lower cholesterol through diet—

but only as long as they are substituted for other fats, not used in addition to them.

VERY-LOW-FAT DIETS

If reducing the fat in your diet a little is good for you, wouldn't reducing the fat in your diet a lot be even better? It sounds logical, but in reality, very-low-fat diets don't help your health much in the short run, and in the long run they may even be damaging.

Two very-low-fat diets have gotten a lot of media attention. The Ornish diet, created by Dr. Dean Ornish, provides only 7 percent of calories from fat. The Ornish program for treating heart disease combines a very-low-fat, vegetarian diet with moderate exercise, smoking cessation, weight loss, and training in stress reduction. Controlled experiments as part of the Lifestyle Heart Trial, in which heart patients follow the Ornish program, have shown that program participants do show a detectable improvement in their blocked coronary arteries. Their heart arteries open wider and blood flow to the heart improves.[8] More important, after five years, the arteries of the Ornish patients were still open, while the arteries of similar patients following standard medical treatment had closed up even more.[9] Because the Ornish program involves so many lifestyle changes, however, the improvement can't be attributed to the low-fat part of the diet alone. Also, the results of the studies are based on a very small number of patients who received intensive support.

The well-known Pritikin Longevity program for heart patients uses a very-low-fat, high-carbohydrate diet (less than 10 percent of calories from fat) in combination with vigorous exercise. A study in 1997 concluded that combining the Pritikin approach with cholesterol-lowering drugs led to large and rapid reductions in total cholesterol, LDL cholesterol, and triglycerides in the patients—total cholesterol fell on average by 19 percent.[10] As with the Ornish program, the effect of the very-low-fat part of the Pritikin diet can't be separated from the other parts of the program. Based on the current evidence, it's impossible to say that a very-low-fat diet alone helps heart health. In the long term, these diets are very restrictive and hard to live with, even for patients motivated by severe heart disease. So far the only way the patients in the studies seem to manage is with intensive support. For now, authorities such as the American Heart Association don't recommend very-low-fat diets.

FAT-BLOCKING DRUGS

One of the best ways to reduce your cholesterol level is to lose weight if you are obese. Doctors often recommend cutting fat from the diet as a way to cut calories (1 gram of fat has 9 calories, compared to 4 calories per gram of protein or carbohydrates). To help speed weight loss along for severely obese patients, doctors sometimes also prescribe the fat-blocking drug orlistat (Xenical®). This drug, approved by the FDA in 1999, blocks an enzyme in the digestive system and keeps your body from absorbing about a third of the fat you eat. When used with a low-calorie, low-fat diet, orlistat has been shown to help patients lose more weight than with diet alone.

This drug is generally prescribed for people who are severely obese, because it can have unpleasant side effects, including loose stools and anal leakage. Orlistat won't help reduce high blood cholesterol. It works for weight loss only if you also follow a strict diet, and even then it may not be much help.

Chitosan, a dietary supplement derived from shellfish, is promoted as a fat-binding substance that helps you lose weight. When taken with meals, chitosan is said to bind to fatty acids in the stomach and to prevent their absorption in the intestines. There's not a lot of evidence to show that chitosan is effective.

BEYOND DIET

Even if you eat oatmeal for breakfast faithfully every day, use a cholesterol-lowering spread, and follow every other dietary suggestion to lower your cholesterol, you will probably only be able to reduce your LDL cholesterol by about 10 percent. To get your LDL cholesterol below the recommended level, diet alone might not be enough. Also, the beneficial effects of improving your diet don't happen overnight—they take a good two years to be fully felt. If you're at risk of heart disease, then, there's a good chance your doctor will recommend one of the cholesterol-lowering statin drugs such as lovastatin (Mevacor®), simvastatin (Zocor®), or atorvastatin (Lipitor®). These drugs can reduce LDL cholesterol levels by as much as 30 percent, and they do help prevent heart attacks. So far, all the studies suggest they work well, but some people experience side effects, such as liver problems and muscle pain. And so far no studies can say whether taking these drugs for decades will really prolong your life or even be safe in the long run.

What's the bottom line? First, see your doctor and get your blood lipids checked. Be sure to do this after fasting for at least twelve hours—otherwise, your triglycerides reading may not be accurate. Your cholesterol levels have a certain amount of normal variation from day to day. A borderline high reading one day could be normal or even slightly below normal a few days later, so if you come in on the high side, repeat the test a week or so later before making any decisions about medication. If your cholesterol really is too high, there are many steps that, in combination, may bring it down to a better level without drugs: lose weight, stop smoking, exercise more, reduce your dietary cholesterol, try a cholesterol-lowering margarine, and eat more fiber.

Chapter Five
TAKING OUT THE TRANS FATS

It's pretty clear that trans fats aren't good for you. It's also pretty clear that eating less of them is a good idea. Good as the idea might be, however, putting it into action is more difficult. What makes trans fats so hard to avoid is that they're everywhere. Today trans fats are found in almost all baked goods, processed and packaged foods, and snack foods. Even foods that claim to be healthful, like granola bars, turn out to be loaded not just with sugar but with trans fats. Not surprisingly, the major sources of trans fats in the American diet are prepared baked goods of every sort, including bread, cookies, crackers, baking mixes, frozen baked goods, and refrigerated bread and pastry products. More unexpectedly, another big source of trans fats is packaged breakfast cereals, especially the sweet ones marketed heavily to children. Chip-type snacks are a major source of trans fats in the diet. The biggest culprits of all, however, are fast-food restaurants. The doughnuts and other baked goods, special sauces and creamy salad dressings, chicken nuggets, fried chicken, fried fish filets, and especially french fries at these places contribute huge amounts of trans fats to the typical American diet.

A typical serving of french fries contains about 7 grams of trans fats, but the restaurants aren't required to tell you about them. Ironically, in 1990 McDonald's responded to public concern about saturated fat in the french fries by switching the fat in the deep fryers from tallow (beef fat) to partially hydrogenated vegetable oil. The switch actually made their fries even less healthful than they were before. Instead of revealing that information, however, McDonald's proudly—and accurately—claims that their fries are cholesterol free. McDonald's is hardly alone—all fast-food chains make the same claims.

Fast-food restaurants are only part of the trans fats problem. According to the FDA, some 42,720 food products on the market today contain partially hydrogenated vegetable oil; in almost every category, at least 70 percent of those products contain at least 0.5 grams of trans fat per serving. In the cookies and crackers categories, 100 percent of the products contain more than 0.5 grams of trans fats per serving—every single one of 7,500 products. Among the baking needs (pie shells, frostings, chocolate chips, and similar products), the total is also 100 percent.

Overall, of those 42,720 products, 31,930 contain at least 0.5 grams of trans fat per serving. It's a grim picture, one that goes a long way toward explaining why over a third of all Americans are seriously overweight and why nearly 35 million of them have high cholesterol levels.

TRANS FATS IN YOUR DIET

Just how many grams of trans fats are you eating every day? The answer to that is a little controversial, because it depends a lot on who you ask and how they count. According to the USDA's Continuing Survey of Food Intake by Individuals (CSFII), the average American takes in 5.3 grams of trans fats a day, or about 2.6 percent of total calories.[1]

That number is probably on the low side, though. The FDA has calculated a somewhat higher number based on more recent CSFII information. According to the FDA, the average adult male takes in 7.62 grams of trans fats a day, or nearly 3 percent of his total calories. The average female takes in 5.54 grams of trans fats, or just over 3 percent of her total calories. On average, adult Americans are getting 2.91 percent of their daily calories from trans fats.[2] Given the powerful negative effect trans fats have on your cholesterol, how much is safe to eat? Right now, there's no official answer to that question. The unofficial answer from concerned nutritionists and doctors is as little as possible. They suggest that you count your trans fat intake as part of your daily saturated fat intake—something that will become much easier to do once the new labeling requirements are in place.

The Department of Health in the United Kingdom has had an official recommendation since 1994. Here's what they say: "We recommend that, on average, trans fatty acids should provide no more than the current average of about 2% of dietary energy and consideration should be given to ways of decreasing the amount present in the diet."[3]

For a typical 2,000-calorie diet, 2 percent of dietary energy works out to 4.4 grams of trans fat daily.

The current American average intake of trans fats is 5 grams a day, pretty close to the average amount in the United Kingdon. You definitely don't want your intake to be any higher—and lower would be better. According to the dietary guidelines, your total daily intake of all fats should be no more than 30 percent of total calories, and saturated fat intake should be 8 to 10 percent of your total calories. In practical terms, that means limiting your saturated and trans fats to about 20 to 25 grams daily. Given that trans fats are about twice as deadly as saturated fat, however, it makes sense to keep your intake as low as possible, preferably well under 5 grams a day.

To lower your trans fat intake to 5 grams a day or less probably means that you'll have to give up many of the baked goods, fast foods, and processed foods that are so much a part of the American diet. A single doughnut at breakfast has about 3 grams of trans fats; a large serving of french fries at lunch has nearly 7 grams. Add them up and you're already at nearly 10 grams of trans fats—twice the 5 grams you're aiming for and also nearly half of your total saturated/trans fat allowance for the day. And those 10 grams are in addition to the almost unavoidable trans fats in all the other foods you might eat in a day.

Some manufacturers use wording on their packaging that could fool you into eating more trans fats than you realize. Labels that proclaim the food has no cholesterol or is cooked in 100 percent vegetable oil are very misleading. Trans fats are made from plant oils, so by definition they don't have any cholesterol and are vegetable oils. If the food has been cooked in vegetable oil, it's a near certainty that the oil was partially hydrogenated. This sort of misleading labeling will become obsolete when the new trans fat labeling rule comes into effect.

THE FAST-FOOD TRANS TRAP

A recent study based on the CSFII data looked at the amounts and types of vegetables American children eat. The researchers at Pennington Biomedical Research Institute in Louisiana found that just two foods—french fries and potato chips—made up about a third of the vegetables. (Believe it or not, the U.S. Department of Agriculture classifies potato chips as a vegetable—which means, among other things, that potato chips officially count as vegetables in school lunches.) Among children aged six and under, 27.3 percent of their vegetables came from these two potato products; in the seven- to twelve-year age group, 28.9 percent came from chips and fries; and in the thirteen- to eighteen-year age group, these two potato products made up 31.2 percent of their total vegetables. Among African American children in the thirteen- to eighteen-year age group, the number went up to 40 percent. Adults aged nineteen to thirty don't do much better: Potato chips and french fries made up 22 to 25 percent of total vegetable consumption.[4] And a recent survey by the World Health Organization found that 31 percent of American fifteen-year-olds ate french fries every day.[5]

Today the typical American eats over 30 pounds of french fries every year, up from about 4 pounds a year in 1960. Nearly 90 percent of those fries are purchased at fast-food restaurants.[6] One reason kids eat so many fries is that many American schools have meal contracts with fast-food restaurants to bring the fries right into the lunchroom.

With such poor nutrition being actively encouraged by the schools, to say nothing of the huge amount of advertising the fast-food chains direct at children, it's hardly surprising that a third of all American children are overweight and one in five is obese. What's worse, the high trans fats content of these nutritionally worthless foods are setting these kids up for early heart disease. A medium serving of french fries has about 17 grams of fat, including about 7 grams of saturated fat and 7 of trans fats. Depending on the brand, a serving of potato chips has roughly 30 grams of fat, including 10 grams of saturated fat and about 3 grams of trans fats. Predictably, 60 percent of overweight children and teens already have at least one risk factor for heart disease, such as raised blood pressure.[7]

SNACKING ON TRANS FATS

One-third of the American diet today consists of junk food. That means high-calorie (and usually high-fat), low-nutrient, highly processed foods that don't belong to any of the five major food groups: dairy, fruit, grains, meat and beans, and vegetables. Recent research shows that the average American adult gets 27 percent of his or her total daily calories from junk foods and an additional 4 percent from alcoholic beverages. About 33 percent of Americans get an average of 45 percent of their calories from these empty foods.[8]

Kids today eat twice as many snack foods as they did in the late 1970s. They now take in about 25 percent of their daily calories from snacks, mostly crackers, popcorn, pretzels, and corn chips. As the amount of snack food in kids' diets increases, the amount of fruit, vegetables, and milk in their diet drops. Overall, nearly two-thirds of American children are not getting the recommended amounts of vitamin E and zinc in their diets; half don't get enough calcium; and nearly a third don't get enough iron and vitamin B_6.

What kids today are getting plenty of is trans fats. Sweet baked snacks, such as cookies, are high in trans fats, but salty snacks, such as crackers and chips, are even higher—and the consumption of salty, high-fat snacks has doubled over the past 20 years or so.[9] All these worthless foods are not only high in trans fats, they displace higher-quality foods from the diet, leaving kids and adults short on vitamins, minerals, fiber, and everything else that goes into healthy eating.

MARGARINE VS. BUTTER

Americans may not know that french fries are bad for their hearts, but they're convinced that eating margarine instead of butter is good for them. They're wrong. The average American gets anywhere from 25 to 37 percent of his or her daily dose of trans fats from margarine. (A small part of this may come from butter, which naturally contains a very small amount of trans fats.)[10] If you want to cut your trans fat intake, eliminating margarine would be a good place to start.

For decades now, the vegetable oil industry and health professionals have advised people to use margarine instead of butter. All that advice has paid off: Today per capita consumption of margarine in the United States is 8.3 pounds, while butter consumption is down to about 4.2 pounds. The evidence suggests, however, that margarine is no healthier than butter—and, in fact, it may be worse. To take just one example, a 1997 study in the journal *Epidemiology* looked at the heart disease levels among participants in the Framingham Health Study. This ongoing study followed the diet, lifestyle, and health of a large group of men living near Boston. In the late 1960s, when margarine was first being touted as good for the heart, the researchers asked the Framingham men how much margarine they ate each day. Based on the answers and follow-up over the next twenty-one years, the researchers discovered that the more margarine a participant ate, the *more likely* he was to develop heart disease, even when factors like smoking and obesity were taken into account. The researchers found that margarine intake turned out to be a good predictor of future heart trouble. They also found that butter intake was not a predictor: The Framingham men who ate a lot of butter didn't have predictably higher rates of heart disease later in life.[11]

A number of dietary trials over the years have compared the effects of butter and margarine on cholesterol level. Recently researchers in the Netherlands did a meta-analysis of the studies—they looked at them all and used powerful statistical tools to analyze the results. Their results were unequivocal. Replacing butter with hard stick margarine—which usually contains anywhere from 20 to 25 percent trans fats—has no effect at all on your cholesterol level. Replacing butter with soft tub margarine, which is lower in trans fats, has a slight lowering effect on LDL cholesterol, but does nothing to raise HDL cholesterol.[12] The conclusion? In the words of researchers at the Harvard School of Public Health: "[I]ndividuals who are replacing butter with margarine high in trans fat to reduce their risks of coronary disease may obtain no benefit or—if trans fat has deleterious effects beyond those on LDL and HDL—may even increase their risk."[13]

On the other hand, a recent study showed that tub margarine containing only 7 percent trans fat does help reduce LDL cholesterol, at least for some people. It doesn't seem to help overweight people as much as normal-weight people. There's also a fair amount of variation among individuals, which suggests that the response is at least in part genetically based. Margarine had no effect on HDL cholesterol.

The study is scientifically sound, but note that the work was funded by the United Soybean Board and the National Association of Margarine Manufacturers along with the General Clinical Research Center at the University of Texas Southwestern Medical Center.[14]

The American Heart Association still recommends using margarine instead of butter. The thinking behind this is that butter contains a lot more saturated fat than margarine as well as 31 mg of cholesterol per tablespoon. In addition, margarine contains polyunsaturated vegetable oil, which may help lower cholesterol. Even so, the AHA's most recent medical/scientific statement on the subject suggests you choose soft margarines over harder, stick forms and recommends choosing a brand with no more than 2 grams of saturated fat per tablespoon and with liquid vegetable oil as the first ingredient.[15] You'll have to decide for yourself if you want to continue using margarine instead of butter. Some margarine manufacturers have begun making liquid or soft spreads with reduced or no trans fats, but most still contain plenty. Check the fat counter in the back of this book for a breakdown of the trans fats ranges for butter and the different types of margarines.

MARGARINE ALTERNATIVES

Cholesterol-lowering margarines made with plant sterols and no trans fats are now on the market. A number of new margarines and spreads made without trans fats are now available as well.

Among the spreads are Spectrum Naturals®, which are made using vegetable oils and natural gums as the thickening agent. Smart Balance® spread, developed by nutrition experts at Brandeis University, is made with a blend of four oils: soy, canola, olive, and palm. The spread contains the same proportions of poly, mono, and saturated fats recommended by the American Heart Association. Trans fat–free margarines still have calories and fat—most check in at about 80 calories and 10 grams of total fat per tablespoon.

Among the margarine brands, Promise Ultra Fat-Free®, Smart Beat Fat-Free Squeeze®, and Fleischmann's Fat-Free Spread® are free of all fats, including trans fats. Promise Spread® has no trans fats, but it's not fat free. The fat-free spreads are lower in calories, ranging from 5 to 50 calories or even more per tablespoon.

All the trans fat–free and fat-free margarines are very soft—they're meant to be used only as spreads and toppings. Don't use them for cooking or baking.

FINDING THE HIDDEN TRANS FATS

Most manufacturers have never analyzed their products for trans fats, mostly because until very recently it wasn't a government requirement, as the total fat and saturated fat counts were. The new trans fat labeling requirement will take several years to go into full effect. In the meantime, the table in the back of this book lists the trans fat content for those foods that have been analyzed. The information comes from the U.S. Department of Agriculture and from the Harvard School of Public Health.

Where the trans fat content isn't known, you can make an educated guess. If the ingredients label lists hydrogenated or partially hydrogenated vegetable oil as an ingredient, the product contains trans fats, no matter how healthy the manufacturer claims it is. The closer the partially hydrogenated vegetable oil is to the top of the ingredients list, the more the food contains.

You can estimate the trans fat content of a food by looking at the total fat content per portion and subtracting the saturated fat, monounsaturated fat, and polyunsaturated fat. The difference is the trans fat content. It's often a very small number—0.5 grams or less. In many cases, because manufacturers are allowed to round the fat grams, the sum of all the fats matches the total fat, even when the product contains trans fats. But even small amounts of trans fat add up, because they're twice as bad for you as saturated fat. Half a gram of trans fat is about equal in artery-clogging power to 1 gram of saturated fat.

Unfortunately, until the new FDA regulation on trans fats goes into effect, the food label is required to list only the total fat and the saturated fat; in most cases, no other fats are mentioned. You still can get a rough idea of the trans fat in the food. A good rule of thumb is that if saturated fat is only a small portion of the total fat content—say 3 grams out of 9—the food is almost certainly high in trans fats and should be avoided if possible.

Fast foods and restaurant foods are exempt from the federal food labeling requirements, so it's almost impossible to know the trans fat content of the foods you eat when you go out. That's a big problem, because today most Americans eat at least one meal a day away from home—and that meal is very likely to be in a fast-food restaurant. The fast-food chains will provide nutritional information at the restaurant if you ask, and some post the information on their websites, but they don't break out the trans fat content. They do provide the total fat and saturated fat content, however, so here, too, it's possible to make an informed estimate of the trans fats in a food item.

AVOIDING TRANS FATS

It's probably impossible and not really necessary to avoid trans fats in your diet completely. It's a very good idea, however, to cut down on them as much as possible. Even though trans fats are very widely used in our foods, you can reduce your consumption without too much trouble. In fact, you can even enjoy a meal in a fast-food restaurant if you choose carefully.

Start by cutting back on snacking. All those cookies,

cakes, potato chips, tortilla chips, corn chips, and other junk foods are full of trans fats and empty of nutrition. Substitute healthier snacks such as fresh or dried fruits, carrot sticks and other vegetables, cheese, or no-fat pretzels. Try home-made air-popped popcorn with butter or some trans fat–free liquid spread instead of butter-flavored microwave pop-corn—the "butter" is really flavored partially hydrogenated vegetable oil. A typical serving of butter-flavored microwave popcorn has 2.2 grams of trans fats.

Next, cut back on your home use of prepared and highly processed foods, especially packaged or frozen deep-fried foods. Fried chicken, french fries, hashed browns, potato puffs, fish sticks, tacos (the shells are fried), mozzarella sticks, and the like are all prepared using trans fats and lots of them. Read labels carefully—if partially hydrogenated vegetable oil is in the top five ingredients, avoid the product. Look for healthier entrees and side dishes that are baked, sauteed, or steamed. Even then, however, check that label. These products can still be high in trans fats.

The hardest step is cutting back on prepared baked goods. The sweeter the product, the more trans fats it proba-bly contains, in order to maintain its texture and moisture. Doughnuts are high in trans fats; cookies and cakes aren't too far behind. Muffins, Danish pastry, and sweet rolls are also high in trans fats; so are toaster pastries. Most breads have some trans fats, but the amount is considerably less than for the sweeter products. Mixes for homemade cookies, cakes, pancakes, and breads all contain partially hydro-genated vegetable oil. So do refrigerated dough products for cookies, rolls, and biscuits. Trans fats are even in many cold breakfast cereals—the sweeter the cereal, the more likely it is to contain trans fats.

It's hard to cut back on these foods, because so many of them are eaten at breakfast, on coffee breaks, or as snacks. Start by aiming for a healthier breakfast—you'll lose some trans fats and probably some weight, as well. Switch to unsweetened cereals such as corn flakes or oatmeal or try a toasted pita or English muffin instead of a toaster pastry. If you like to cook, make your own quick breads and muffins and freeze them in individual portions. It's healthier and far less expensive than toaster pastries, mixes, or refrigerated dough.

Try to cut back on some of the less obvious sources of trans fats. Prepared mayonnaise, for instance, contains trans fats. Many prepared salad dressing are high in trans fats, especially the creamy ones. Ramen noodles and many "instant" noodle products turn out to be high in trans fats—the noodles are fried as part of the process that makes them cook so quickly.

When it comes to eating out, especially in fast-food restaurants, choose carefully. Skip anything deep-fried, especially chicken nuggets or fried chicken, avoid the french fries, and don't eat the cookies or fruit-filled pastries. A few chains offer baked potatoes as an alternative to the inevitable french fries. Some restaurant chains offer a reasonable choice of salads, but be careful here—the packaged salad dressings are usually high in trans fats. All those creamy dressings—creamy Italian, ranch, Caesar, Thousand Island—are high in saturated fat and trans fats.

There's no question that cutting back on trans fats isn't easy—after all, we eat so many fried foods and potato chips because they taste good. Cutting back doesn't mean eliminating. If you have french fries as an occasional treat instead of eliminating them entirely, you'll enjoy them even more. At the same time, you'll be eating a better diet that will pay off in healthier arteries and a lower chance of heart disease.

Chapter Six
FATS AND THE FOOD LABEL

The federal Food and Drug Administration requires all packaged foods to have a nutrition facts panel on the food label. This is a convenient source of important information about the fat content of the food. By checking the label carefully and understanding the slightly confusing standards it uses, you can get a pretty good idea of the total fat, saturated fat, and cholesterol content. And once the proposed new FDA labeling requirements for trans fats are in place, you'll also be able to learn how much of this killer fat is in the food.

To understand the food label, start by looking at the top, where the serving size and the number of servings in the package are listed—all the information that follows will assume that you will eat only one serving of the usual size. The portion sizes are smaller than you might think. Be realistic when deciding how the food fits into your daily goal of only 30 grams of fat. The portion size for cookies, for instance, might be just one. Will you really be eating just one cookie?

Next on the list are the calories per serving and the calories from fat. This is pretty self-explanatory, but the next section of the label, the nutrients content, can be a bit confusing. (On many products this section of the label is now in yellow.) The first items in this part are the nutrients that Americans generally eat in more than adequate amounts: fat, cholesterol, and sodium (salt). The purpose of giving the information about these nutrients is so that you can limit them in your diet.

The first item on this part of the list is the total fat per serving. Under the total fat content is the saturated fat content. For some products, such as vegetable oils, the list also provides the monounsaturated and polyunsaturated fat content. (This is a requirement only where the amounts of mono and poly fat are considered relevant, and it doesn't usually show up on the label.)

The next item on the list is the cholesterol content of the food, even if it doesn't have any.

The amounts for fats are given in grams. (A gram is 1,000 milligrams, or about ¼ teaspoon or 0.035 of an ounce.) The amounts for cholesterol are given in milligrams (abbreviated mg). Both fat and cholesterol also are given as a percentage of the recommended daily amounts for adults, officially called the Percent Daily Value (abbreviated as %DV). On labels that are large enough, the %DV is followed by an asterisk. This leads you to a short explanation at the bottom of the label that reads "*Percent Daily Values are based on a 2,000 calorie diet. Your Daily Values may be higher or lower depending on your calorie needs." If the label is big enough, following that explanation is a chart of the Percent Daily Values. An optional footnote for packages of any size is the number of calories per gram of fat (9) and carbohydrate and protein (4 each).

The Percent Daily Value assumes you eat 2,000 calories a day, about average for an adult, that 30 percent of those calories should come from fat, and that 10 percent should come from saturated fat.

Another way to look at the %DV is as a scale for estimating your total daily fat intake. If the %DV for fat of a portion is 15 percent, for instance, then you know that you still have 85 percent of your daily intake to go (100 percent minus 15 percent is 85 percent).

Even if you don't keep track of your daily calories or fat grams, you still can use the %DV as a handy frame of reference. It's also helpful for comparison purposes if you want to choose a product or brand with the lowest fat content. You also can use the %DV to figure out some fat trade-offs. If you eat a food that's high in fat, you can balance it out with lower-fat foods—just aim to keep the total amount of fat for the day at or below 100 percent of the Daily Value.

Until the new trans fat label regulation comes into effect, there is one glaring problem with the %DV for fat: Trans fats are not included. Consumers today know they should select foods that are low in saturated fat. But when those foods are low in saturated fats and high in trans fats, health-conscious consumers are unknowingly jumping out of the frying pan and into the deep fryer. Fortunately, this misleading situation will be corrected by the new FDA trans fat labeling requirement.

FATS FOR KIDS

Special rules apply to the labels on food for kids under age four. The label provides the Percent Daily Values for vitamins, minerals, and protein, because they have been established for kids in that age group, but it doesn't contain this information for the fat, fiber, and sodium content, because those %DVs haven't been established. There's another reason as well: Kids need fat, and plenty of it, in their diet in order to grow properly. The FDA believes that listing a %DV for fat in baby foods wrongly suggests to parents that fat for children should be limited. (There are special labeling requirements for infant formulas.)

LET THERE BE LITE

Products that proclaim they have less fat are now strictly regulated by the FDA. Here's what the nutrient content claims mean:

• **Free.** The product contains no amount, or only trace amounts, of one or more of these components: fat, saturated fat, cholesterol, sodium, sugars, and calories. For example, fat-free means there is less than 0.5 mg of fat per serving. Synonyms for free include "without," "no," and "zero."

• **Low.** This term can be used on foods that can be eaten frequently without exceeding the guidelines for one or more of these components: fat, saturated fat, cholesterol, sodium, and calories. "Low fat" means the food has 3 grams or less per serving; "low saturated fat" means the food has 1 gram or less per serving; "low cholesterol" means the food has 20 milligrams or less of cholesterol *and* 2 grams or less of saturated fat per serving. Synonyms for low include "little," "few," "low source of," and "contains a small amount of."

• **Reduced.** This means the product has been altered to contain at least 25 percent less of a nutrient or calories than the regular product. If the regular product already meets the "low" claim, however, the manufacturer can't make the reduced claim.

• **Less.** The food, whether altered or not, contains 25 percent less of nutrient or calories than a reference product. For example, a manufacturer can claim that its pretzels have 25 percent less fat than a rival's potato chips. "Fewer" is a synonym for less.

• **Light or lite.** The food has been altered to contain half the fat or one-third fewer calories than the regular product.

• **Percent fat free.** If a manufacturer wants to make this claim, the product must be low fat or fat free. The claim must be based on 100 grams of the food. So, if a food contains 2.5 grams of fat per 50 grams (5 grams of fat per 100 grams), the label can claim the food is "95 percent fat free."

• **Lean and extra lean.** These terms are used to describe the fat content of meat, poultry, and seafood. Lean means the food has less than 10 grams of fat, 4.5 grams or less of saturated fat, and less than 95 milligrams of cholesterol per serving and per 100 grams. Extra lean means the food has less than 5 grams of fat, 2 grams or less of saturated fat, and less than 95 milligrams of cholesterol per serving and per 100 grams.

Pretty confusing, isn't it? If you can't remember all these definitions (who except a government bureaucrat could?), just remember to check the Percent Daily Value for fat and saturated fat. The lower the numbers, the better.

When a label proclaims that the product has no cholesterol, it can still be bad for you in other ways. Cholesterol is found only in animal foods, so anything that doesn't contain animal fat is by definition cholesterol free. In other words, cookies that don't contain cholesterol don't contain any butter—but they do contain plenty of trans fats instead. They're not any more healthful—in fact, because of the trans fat content, they're less healthful than cookies made with real butter.

THE MILK LABEL

A lot of adults, and far too many kids and teenagers, don't drink milk. They think it has too many calories and too much fat, so they drink nutritionally empty diet (and often caffeine-laden) sodas instead. These people are sadly misinformed. They're losing out on an excellent—and low-fat—source of nutrition. The labeling requirements for milk were changed in 1998 to make them more accurate (or maybe just to confuse consumers about what exactly skim milk is). Here's what to look for:

- **Fat-free milk.** Contains 0 grams of fat and 80 calories per 8 fluid ounces (1 cup). Also known as skim milk or nonfat milk.

- **Low-fat milk.** Contains 3 grams of fat or less and 100 calories per 8 fluid ounces (1 cup). Also known as ½% or 1% milk.

- **Reduced-fat milk.** Contains at least 25 percent less fat than whole milk; generally contains 5 grams of fat and 120 calories per 8 fluid ounces (1 cup). Also known as 2% milk.

- **Whole milk.** Contains 8 grams of fat and 150 calories per 8 fluid ounces (1 cup).

The good thing about the lower-fat milks is that they all still have the same 300 milligrams of calcium found in 8 ounces of whole milk. That's about a quarter of your daily requirement of 1,000 to 1,200 milligrams. Department of Agriculture studies have shown that most adult women and many children don't meet the daily requirement for calcium. Don't let fear of fat keep you from getting your calcium from the best natural source—the latest evidence shows that regular milk drinkers have no increased risk of heart disease. In fact, a recent study shows that men who drink one to two cups of milk a day have an 8 percent lower risk of death from heart disease; their risk of death from all causes, including cancer and stroke, is 10 percent lower.[1]

STAKING CLAIMS

The FDA recently has started allowing food manufacturers to make some kinds of health claims on the package labeling. Here's what the FDA allows food manufacturers to say about dietary fat:

  • **Cancer.** "Development of cancer depends on many factors. A diet low in total fat may reduce the risk of some cancers."

  • **Coronary heart disease.** "While many factors affect heart disease, diets low in saturated fat and cholesterol may reduce the risk of this disease."

The claim can be made only if the food meets the definition for low fat, low saturated fat, low cholesterol, or extra lean.

In general, foods that make health claims are low in fat and cholesterol and high in nutrients that are important for heart health, such as fiber, folic acid, and potassium.

THE TRANS FAT LABEL

In November 1999 the FDA proposed a new food labeling rule that would require the amounts of trans fatty acids present in a food to be listed. The amount would be included in the amount and Percent Daily Value (%DV) of saturated fat by adding an asterisk to the saturated fat numbers. The asterisk would refer consumers to a footnote at the bottom of the

nutrition label that would give the number of grams of trans
fats in each serving.

In addition to proposing that the amount of trans fats be
listed on the food label, the FDA also has proposed that
wherever saturated fat limits are placed on nutrient content
claims or health claims, the trans fat content of the food has
to be taken into account. The FDA has also proposed a new
labeling claim of "trans fat free."

By proposing the new rule, the FDA was responding, in
part, to a citizen petition sponsored by the Center for Sci-
ence in the Public Interest (CSPI), a watchdog group that
has been in the forefront of consumer lobbying for more
healthful foods. The FDA also was responding to the over-
whelming new scientific evidence that trans fats are very un-
healthful. Based on current labeling requirements, a food
could contain more trans fat than saturated fat per serving,
yet consumers would have no way of knowing the real fat
content. The new rule is designed to prevent misleading
claims and to provide the information consumers need to select healthful foods. After all, if you choose a food that that
claims to be low in saturated fat or cholesterol, you should
be confident that the food really is more healthful—and if
it's high in trans fat, it's not, no matter how low it is in other
fats.

The FDA hopes that, over time, the new rule also will
help reduce the incidence of coronary heart disease. It
feels that the rule will have a twofold effect. First, consumers will be able to reduce their intake of trans fats
more easily. Second, food manufacturers will face increased consumer demand for trans fat–free foods and will
reformulate their products to eliminate the partially hydrogenated vegetable oils. In most cases reformulation will
not be particularly difficult or expensive, so it is unlikely
to raise consumer costs even as it improves consumer
health.

From a health standpoint, perhaps the most important as-
pect of the new labeling requirement is that the trans fat con-

tent will be included in the Percent Daily Value (%DV) for saturated fat. This crucial change recognizes that trans fats are just as bad, if not worse, for your arteries than saturated fat. By increasing the %DV for saturated fat, consumers will have a much more accurate idea of how a particular food fits into their fat ration for the day. It also will make consumers far more aware of how quickly the saturated fat in their diet adds up.

THE TRANS FAT–FREE CLAIM

As consumers become more aware of the dangers of trans fats, both from the new labeling rule and from other sources, food producers will want to claim that their products have no trans fats. The new labeling rule provides some guidelines for exactly how the claim can be made.

The trans fat–free claim can be made only if the food has 0.5 g or less of saturated fat per serving *and* 0.5 g or less of trans fats per serving. The reasoning here is consumers reasonably expect a food low in trans fats also to be low in saturated fat.

BENEFITS OF THE NEW LABEL

What if the new label was so effective that all food manufacturers reformulated their products to eliminate trans fats? That's a pretty unlikely scenario, but even so, researchers have calculated what would happen to heart disease rates if it happened. Depending on how you look at the numbers, in ten years' time the nationwide risk of coronary heart disease would drop anywhere from 4.28 to 8.36 percent.

Realistically speaking, the FDA figures on a more likely scenario: Some manufacturers will reformulate their products, and some consumers will cut back on products that contain trans fat. If all manufacturers reformulated their margarines to remove the trans fat, and if 3 percent of the breads and cakes and 15 percent of the cookies and crackers were reformulated to remove the trans fat, in ten years the result still would be highly beneficial.

This scenario is quite plausible: In Germany and some other European countries, trans fat labeling requirements have led all margarine manufacturers to reformulate their products to eliminate partially hydrogenated vegetable oils. Because of increased consumer awareness, at least 30 percent of the margarines on the market in the United States already have no trans fat.

The FDA estimates that, overall, Americans would reduce their intake of trans fat by about 1 percent simply by knowing which products contain it and avoiding or eating less of them. When that happens, the risk of coronary heart disease nationwide will drop by somewhere between 0.86 and 1.67 percent.

That may not seem like a big reduction, but it is when you work out the numbers. The American Heart Association estimates that every year Americans have 1.1 million heart attacks caused by coronary heart disease—and a third of those heart attacks are fatal.

Even the modest decrease in trans fat intake the FDA predicts from the new labeling requirement will lead to a significant drop in heart disease and death. According to FDA studies, removing trans fats from all margarine would prevent approximately 6,300 heart attacks, including 2,100 deaths, each year. Additionally, removing trans fats from 3 percent of breads and cakes and 15 percent of cookies and crackers would prevent an estimated 17,100 heart attacks, including 5,600 deaths, each year.[2]

The savings in dollar terms are enormous. The American Heart Association estimates that the total annual cost of nonfatal coronary heart disease comes out to some $51.1 *billion*.[3] The FDA estimates that three years after the new trans fat labeling requirement goes into effect, the annual cost savings will be at least $2.9 billion and could be as high as $7.9 billion. Over twenty years, the estimated savings in healthcare costs would be somewhere between $25 billion and $59 billion.

Chapter Seven
THE GOOD FATS

It should be pretty clear by now that the less saturated a fat is, the better it is for your health. It makes good heart sense, then, to substitute unsaturated fats for saturated fats and trans fats. But as you'll learn in this chapter, the good fats help more than just your heart.

MUFAS AND PUFAS

Monounsaturated fatty acids (MUFAs) and polyunsaturated fatty acids (PUFAs) are oils—fats that are liquid at room temperature.

There are several different kinds of MUFAs, but the one that's most common in the diet is oleic acid, the main fat in olive oil.

There are also a number of different kinds of PUFAs. In general, vegetable oils such as corn oil or canola oil are good dietary sources of PUFAs; there are also PUFAs in animal fat, eggs, and fish, and in nuts, seeds, and dark-green leafy vegetables. Two kinds of polyunsaturated fat, linoleic acid and linolenic acid, are known as essential fatty acids, or EFAs. To maintain good health, you must get sufficient amounts of both these fatty acids from your diet.

MONOUNSATURATED FATS AND YOUR HEALTH

When it comes to your health, the most important monounsaturated fatty acid is oleic acid, the main fatty acid in olive oil. Oleic acid is also found in abundance in nuts, including almonds, cashews, hazelnuts, macadamia, peanuts, pecans, and pistachios. (Technically, peanuts are legumes, but in any discussion of MUFA they can be classified as nuts.) Other dietary sources of oleic acid are avocados, canola oil, peanut oil, and, in smaller amounts, animal fats and butter. Also, because oleic acid is found in the cell membranes of plants, you get some oleic acid from eating fruits, vegetables, and whole grains.

For most people, the primary source of oleic acid in the diet fat is olive oil. About 80 percent of olive oil is made up of monounsaturated oleic acid; about 8 to 10 percent is linoleic acid; and about 1 percent is linolenic acid. Other monounsaturated oils found widely in the diet are canola oil and peanut oil, both of which have more polyunsaturated fat relative to monounsaturated fat than olive oil. Other vegetable oils contain some monounsaturated fat in the form of oleic acid, but many widely used oils, such as corn oil and safflower oil, contain a greater proportion of polyunsaturated fats to the monounsaturated fat. (Check the fat counter at the back of this book for the fat content of various commonly used vegetable oils.)

OLIVE OIL AND YOUR HEALTH

Although hazelnut oil is a bit higher in MUFA than olive oil, it is quite expensive and has a strong nut flavor. In general, the single best source of monounsaturated fat in the diet is extra-virgin olive oil. This oil is unprocessed and contains the most oleic acid and EFAs. (For more on how olive oil and other vegetable oils are made, and which ones to choose, see Chapter 8.)

Olive oil is flavorful and versatile in the kitchen, but its virtues extend far beyond mere taste. A growing body of scientific evidence shows that monounsaturated fats, and especially olive oil, have definite health advantages that can help protect you against heart disease and some kinds of cancer.

A number of studies have looked at the role of olive oil in preventing breast cancer. Two studies looked at women in Spain; the other two studies looked at women in Greece and Italy. In all four cases, the women who ate the most olive oil as part of a typical Mediterranean diet had the lowest risk of breast cancer.[1] But was the lowered risk of breast cancer due specifically to the oleic acid in the olive oil or to the fact that olive oil is a monounsaturated fat? A 1998 study in Sweden looked at this question. Because olive oil isn't widely used in that country, the women in the study got most of their dietary fat from dairy products, meat, and margarine. Even though they didn't eat a lot of olive oil, the women who ate the most monounsaturated fat from any source had the lowest rate of breast cancer. In agreement with other studies, the Swedish study also showed that the women who had the most polyunsaturated fat in their diet were somewhat more likely to get breast cancer.[2] Bottom line here: Women, especially those at risk of breast cancer, should consider replacing the saturated and polyunsaturated fats in their diet with monounsaturated fats, particularly olive oil, whenever possible.

Olive oil also may be protective against colon cancer. Researchers at the University of Oxford looked at olive oil consumption in twenty-eight different countries around the world and compared that information to the rates of colon cancer. Countries that had high overall rates of olive oil consumption had low overall rates of colon cancer. People in countries with diets that are high in meat and fish and low in fresh fruits and vegetables had the greatest risk of colon cancer, but even in these countries olive oil had a protective effect.[3]

Over the years a number of researchers have looked at the effects on monounsaturated fats and olive oil on high blood pressure. Most of the studies were inconclusive, mostly because other factors, such as other aspects of the diet, confused the results. However, two recent studies have shown that a diet high in monounsaturated fat can indeed help lower high blood pressure. A 1996 study in Spain showed that a diet high in MUFAs, in the form of either olive oil or sunflower oil, can lead to a significant drop in blood pressure among healthy young men, even when nothing else in the diet changes.[4] In an Italian study published in 2001, Italian researchers put some patients with mild high blood pressure on a diet that was low in saturated fat but high in extra-virgin olive oil; they put some other patients on a diet low in saturated fat but rich in sunflower oil, which is high in polyunsaturated fat. The patients on the olive oil diet all saw their blood pressure drop, to the point where some of them no longer needed their medication. The patients in the sunflower oil group didn't see any improvement.[5] The apparent contradiction on the effect of sunflower oil between the Spanish and Italian studies might be because the subjects in the Spanish study didn't have high blood pressure. The evidence for olive oil in both studies is fairly strong, but other factors may be involved. Other dietary approaches to controlling high blood pressure that substitute olive oil and other vegetable oils for saturated fat also seem to work well.

A long series of controlled dietary studies have shown that PUFA- and MUFA-rich diets lower total cholesterol and LDL cholesterol without lowering HDL cholesterol. The first major study was the Leiden Intervention Trial, dating back to the early 1980s. In this study, men with clogged coronary arteries were put on a vegetarian diet high in polyunsaturated fatty acids and low in saturated fat and cholesterol. In about half the patients, the diet slowed the progression of their heart disease.[6]

The most significant studies of the effects of a diet rich in monounsaturated fat come from the well-known Lyon Heart

Study. This is the recent five-year study that proved the heart-healthy benefits of the Mediterranean diet—a diet rich in whole grains, fresh fruits and vegetables, poultry, fish, and olive oil.

THE CANOLA QUESTION

If you don't like the taste of olive oil, or if you want a milder oil to use in cooking, the best choice is canola oil. Canola oil is made from rapeseed, a plant in the mustard family. Because rapeseed isn't a very appealing name, and because vast amounts of the plant are grown in western Canada, the oil is called canola, from the words Canada and oil.

Overall, canola oil has a bit less saturated fat than olive oil. It also has a good ratio of polyunsaturated to monounsaturated fat.

GOING NUTS

Nuts of all sorts are an excellent way to add monounsaturated fatty acids to your diet. Not only are they a delicious and satisfying snack that's high in beneficial fiber, they could lower your risk of heart disease. In fact, results from the Nurses' Health Study have shown that eating as little as 5 ounces of nuts a week could reduce your cardiovascular risk by 30 to 50 percent.[7] To put that into perspective, it takes about 15 whole cashews to make an ounce. Alternatively, think of an ounce of nuts as a small handful.

Overall, at least five large epidemiological studies and eleven clinical studies have shown that nuts of any kind, including peanuts, help your heart. The evidence shows that the benefit comes from the way the monounsaturated fats in nuts lowers your total cholesterol and LDL cholesterol levels.[8] Of all the nuts, however, walnuts seem to be highest in the fatty acids that help.[9] To see which popular nuts are the best source of unsaturated fat, take a look at the table in the back of the book.

EFAS: CHAINS OF GOOD HEALTH

Two kinds of polyunsaturated fatty acids play an extremely important role in your body—so important, in fact, that nutritionists call them essential fatty acids (EFAs). By "essential," they mean your body must have them and can get them only from your food or supplements.

The two EFAs necessary for human health are linolenic acid (LNA) and linoleic acid (LA). Linolenic acid also is sometimes called alpha linolenic acid, or ALA. Technically speaking, linolenic acid also is called an omega-3 or n-3 essential fatty acid. In fact, the terms "LNA" and "omega-3 fatty acid" often are used interchangeably. In the diet, LNA is found mainly in fish and fish oil, eggs, vegetable oils, nuts and seeds, and dark-green leafy vegetables.

There are also two other omega-3 fatty acids, eicosapentaenoic acid (EPA) and docosahexanoic acid (DHA). Found in fish oil, these two fatty acids aren't essential, but they can be very beneficial to your health. They'll be discussed at length in Chapter 8.

For complex technical reasons, linoleic acid is also called an omega-6 or n-6 essential fatty acid. The main dietary sources of LA are vegetable oils, especially canola oil, safflower oil, and soybean oil.

A third fatty acid, known as arachidonic acid (AA), is another kind of omega-6 fatty acid. At one time researchers believed arachidonic acid was also an essential fatty acid, but it turns out that you can manufacture AA in your body from linoleic acid. Actually, you manufacture about twenty different fatty acids in your body from either linoleic or linolenic acid, so you can see why it's so important to make sure you get enough of both in your diet.

Essential fatty acids play a vital role in your health. You need them to build and maintain your cell membranes, to make the membranes of the smaller structures within each cell (such as the nucleus), to help make the oxygen-carrying hemoglobin in your red blood cells, and for normal cell division and maintenance.

You also need EFAs to make eicosanoids, which in turn are needed to make prostaglandins—short-lived, hormone-like substances your body manufactures and uses to regulate many activities. Among other functions, eicosanoids and prostaglandins help control inflammation, pain, and swelling. They also play important roles in regulating your blood pressure, your heart, your kidneys, and your digestive system. Prostaglandins are also important for making hormones, controlling blood clotting, and triggering allergic reactions. Altogether, your body manufactures at least thirty different kinds of prostaglandins with a wide range of functions.

Prostaglandins are a very complex, two-edged sword. Some, for example, cause swelling, while others relieve it. Because you use omega-3 fatty acids to make some kinds of prostaglandins and omega-6 fatty acids to make others, it's possible to alter your prostaglandin levels, and help improve some health problems, by changing your intake of essential fatty acids. But if you're short on essential fatty acids, you might not be able to make prostaglandins—good or bad—efficiently.

HOW MUCH?

Even though linoleic and linolenic fatty acids are essential to life, there's no official recommended daily amount for them as there are for vitamins and some minerals. In general, if you're a healthy adult who's moderately active, experts say you probably need somewhere in the neighborhood of 4 to 6 grams a day of linoleic acid for good health. That would work out to about 2 to 3 percent of your daily calories (assuming you eat 2,000 calories a day). For linolenic acid, the amount needed is about 2.2 grams a day, or about 1 percent of your daily calories.

THE LOW-FAT TRAP

If you cut your daily fat intake to 30 percent of calories or less, you could have a hard time getting enough EFAs from your diet. That's because other fats, such as saturated fat, trans fats, and heavily processed vegetable oils that are low in omega-3 fatty acids, will take up almost all your fat calories. And by cutting fat across the board and not differentiating between good and bad fats, you reduce your consumption of desirable fats even more. By switching to fat-free salad dressing, for example, you lower your overall fat intake, but at the same time you lose the valuable oleic acid and essential fatty acids found in the olive oil and other vegetable oils used in regular dressings. In the long run, this is probably worse for your health, not better.

Even if you do get more than 30 percent of your calories from fat, there's a good likelihood that you'll be getting your EFAs in the wrong proportions. Ideally, the proportions of your intake of omega-6 and omega-3 fatty acids should be about 2.3 to 1—that is, a bit more than twice as much omega-6 as omega-3. In the typical American diet, however, the ratio of omega-6 to omega-3 is far higher, roughly 10.6 to 1. In terms of grams, that works out to about 12 grams or more a day of linoleic and no more than 1.6 grams a day of linolenic acid. The main reason for the imbalance is that in recent years the amount of corn oil, canola oil, and soybean oil in the American diet has increased sharply. These oils have much more omega-6 fatty acids than omega-3 fatty acids. In corn oil, for instance, the ratio is about 60 parts omega-6 to 1 part omega-3; in soybean oil it's about 7 to 1, and canola oil is about 2 to 1. There hasn't been a corresponding increase in the dietary sources of linolenic acid, such as of fish, eggs, nuts, seeds, and dark-green leafy vegetables,[10] so most people today are eating too much omega-6 and not enough omega-3.

The best way to improve your total intake of essential fatty acids and get them into a better balance is to cut out processed foods and eat more of the foods that are naturally rich in these oils: fish, eggs, nuts, olive oil, whole grains, legumes, and fresh fruits and vegetables. These foods turn out to be the basis of the typical Mediterranean diet—and people who regularly eat this sort of diet tend to have a lot less heart disease and somewhat less cancer. It's also possible to improve your EFA ratio by taking supplements.

BETTER HEALTH WITH EFAS

A large and very impressive body of evidence shows that adding omega-3 fatty acids to the diet can have beneficial effects on your health. In particular, omega-3s are very important for heart health. To take an important recent example, evidence from the ongoing Nurses' Health Study shows that women who eat the most omega-3 fatty acids, regardless of the source, have the lowest risk of having a fatal heart attack. In fact, compared to the women who eat the least omega-3s, their risk is cut by more than half.[11]

Essential fatty acids in the diet come from a variety of foods. The best dietary sources are fish, eggs, nuts, seeds, and vegetable oils; whole grains and green leafy vegetables also contain some. Of all the vegetable oils, flaxseed oil is the highest in EFAs.

Most studies of the benefits of essential fatty acids in the diet, however, have focused on fish oil. That's because starting back in the 1950s, researchers noticed that even though the native peoples of Greenland ate almost nothing but fatty fish and seal meat, they had almost no heart disease or strokes caused by blood clots.[12] Why? Because fish and seal meat (seals eat nothing but fish) are very high in omega-3 fatty acids. Clearly, fish oil was having a protective effect on the hearts of these people.

FISH OIL AND YOUR HEART

The beneficial effects of fish oil on your heart are little short of astonishing, whether the oil comes from supplements or from eating oily fish such as salmon, tuna, or sardines. Currently there's no solid evidence that the omega-3 fatty acids found in fish can prevent coronary heart disease or first heart attacks.[13] However, there's a lot of evidence to show that fish protects your heart in other ways, especially if you already have heart disease.[14]

The first important study to show that fish helps the heart came in 1989 from the ongoing Diet and Reinfarction Trial (DART) study. This study looked at men who had already had a heart attack (myocardial infarction, or MI) and studied ways to help them avoid having a second attack, which is not only likely to happen but is also likely to be fatal. Of the 2,033 men in the study, one-third were advised to reduce the fat and saturated fat in their diet (following the AHA Step I diet) and another third were advised to eat more fiber. The final third were advised to eat fatty fish two to three times a week or, if they hated eating fish, to take half a gram of supplemental fish oil daily. The results? Over a two-year period, the low-fat and fiber groups had no significant improvement in their death rate from any cause. The fatty fish group, however, had a remarkable 29 percent reduction in their overall death rate.[15]

The results of the DART study, first published in 1989, were confirmed ten years later by the GISSI study, a long-term Italian study that looked at fish oil supplements for preventing second heart attacks and strokes in over 11,000 patients who had survived one heart attack. The results of this study showed that over three and a half years, the patients who took 1 gram daily of supplemental fish oil had a 30 percent lower risk of death from heart disease and a 20 percent lower risk of death from all causes, including stroke.[16]

Why does fish help people with damaged hearts? Researchers still don't know for sure, but one possible reason is that fish oil may help make your arteries more elastic.[17] Another possibility is the converse: Fish oil may help keep your arteries from constricting.[18] Either way, the fish oil improves the flow of blood through the arteries that nourish your heart and makes an artery-clogging blood clot less likely to happen.

PREVENTING SUDDEN DEATH

Over 250,000 people die every year in the United States from sudden cardiac arrest, also known as cardiac arrhythmia. Over half of all the victims have no earlier symptoms of heart disease. A 1995 study of deaths from sudden cardiac arrest in the Seattle area showed that eating fatty fish just once a week could cut the risk of dying from this form of heart disease by 50 percent.[19] The protective effects of fish shown by the Seattle study were confirmed by results from the long-running Physicians' Health Study, which tracked the diet and health of over 20,000 male doctors over eleven years. When the study looked at how often these men ate fish, the researchers found no correlation between fish consumption and the chances of having a heart attack caused by clogged coronary arteries. The doctors who ate the most fish were just as likely to have a myocardial infarction as those who ate the least.[20] But when the researchers looked at sudden cardiac death caused by heart rhythm problems, they saw a big difference. Doctors who ate just one fish meal a week were 52 percent less likely to die suddenly from cardiac arrest. Overall, these men also had a lower risk of death from all causes.[21] The benefits of fish extend to all ages.

Older people are 44 percent less likely to die from cardiac arrest if they eat at least one serving of fatty fish weekly.[22]

BLOOD LIPIDS

Eating fish or taking fish oil supplements hasn't been shown to help lower high blood cholesterol, but it does help lower triglycerides. Because high triglycerides are a major risk factor for heart disease, and because the combination of low HDL cholesterol and high triglycerides is especially risky, anything that lowers this type of blood lipid can be useful. A number of studies have shown that fish oil supplements in moderate to large doses help lower triglycerides. Some of the studies also suggest that the fish oil raises HDL cholesterol slightly. Other studies, however, have showed that moderate or even low doses of fish oil supplements raise LDL cholesterol levels enough to be worrisome.[23] Balancing this, however, is a recent study that showed how fish oil supplements help sharply improve HDL/triglyceride ratios in postmenopausal women, whether they were also taking hormone replacement therapy (HRT) or not. (A major drawback to HRT is that it usually increases triglyceride levels.) On average, the women in the study saw their triglyceride levels drop by about 26 percent—which translates into a 27 percent drop in their risk of coronary heart disease. Interestingly, in this study the fish oil supplements did not cause an increase in LDL cholesterol.[24]

STROKE PREVENTION

The old saying that fish is brain food has recently taken on a new meaning, thanks to the ongoing Nurses' Health Study at Harvard Medical School. In 2001, an analysis of dietary patterns from the study showed that the women who ate the most fish and omega-3 fatty acids in general had the lowest risk of stroke, particularly of strokes caused by blood clots in an artery of the brain. Women who ate fish once a week had a 22 percent risk reduction; women who ate fish five or more times a week had a whopping 52 percent lower risk.[25]

Why does eating fish help prevent stroke? Quite possibly because the omega-3 fatty acids in fish thin your blood a bit, which helps prevent clotting. Researchers still don't know exactly how fish oil thins your blood, but because blood clots also can cause heart attacks and other problems, it's a promising area of research.

OTHER BENEFITS OF FISH

The heart-healthy benefits of eating fish are pretty well-documented. Eating fish or taking fish oil supplements seems to help a number of other health problems as well, although in some cases the benefits aren't as clear.

- **High blood pressure.** A number of studies have looked at whether taking fish oil supplements can lower high blood pressure. According to a meta-analysis in 1993 that looked at all the studies, the answer is yes—but only if your blood pressure is high to begin with and even then only by a small amount.[26]

- **Cancer prevention.** The omega-3 fatty acids in fish appear to help prevent certain types of cancer. In particular, people who regularly eat fish have lower rates of cancers of the digestive tract, such as cancer of the esophagus and colon.[27] The omega-3 fatty acids in fish, nuts, and grains also may help protect men against prostate cancer. A 1999 study in the Netherlands showed that the men who ate the most omega-3s had the least risk of prostate cancer.[28] A study of Swedish men in 2001 showed that the ones who never ate fish had a risk of prostate cancer that was two to three times greater than the risk for men who ate fish once or twice a week or more.[29]

• **Rheumatoid arthritis.** This painful disease, quite different from ordinary wear-and-tear osteoarthritis, sometimes responds well to large doses (3 grams a day or more) of fish oil. Researchers still don't know why, although they think the EPA and DHA in fish oil block the production of some inflammatory prostaglandins.[30] If you have rheumatoid arthritis, don't start taking fish oil on your own—discuss it with your doctor first. You'll probably still have to take your anti-inflammatory drugs, but you might be able to reduce the doses.

There have been so many studies showing how fish and fish oil help other health problems that there's no room to go into them all here. Suffice it to say that at least some reputable studies back up the claims that eating fish or taking fish oil supplements helps prevent osteoporosis, helps treat the symptoms of inflammatory bowel disease, helps stabilize the moods of people with bipolar depression, helps prevent premature delivery in at-risk women, and helps prevent age-related macular degeneration (the leading cause of blindness in older adults).

FISH OR FISH OIL?

The evidence in favor of eating fish is so strong that in 1996, the American Heart Association revised its dietary guidelines to specifically recommend fish. Here's how the recommendation reads: "The American Heart Association encourages the consumption of fish as both an excellent source of omega-3 fatty acids and as a good protein source that is low in saturated fat."

The AHA suggests one to two servings of fatty fish per week. Fortunately for fish haters, the bulk of the evidence suggests that all you need is two 4-ounce servings a week to give you the benefits—there's nothing to show that eating fish more often helps your heart even more. To put the fish servings in perspective, a standard can of tuna holds 6 ounces.

Fish oil supplements are more controversial. Is it better to eat more fish or take supplements? Nobody really knows. Most of the studies showing that omega-3 fatty acids help your heart are based on eating fish; only the GISSI study mentioned earlier used fish oil supplements. When fish oil supplements are used to treat problems such as rheumatoid arthritis, the large amount needed can cause heartburn, bloating, gas, diarrhea, and an unpleasant fishy breath and body odor. (The side effects can be avoided at least in part by taking enteric-coated fish oil capsules, which don't re-lease the oil until the capsules reach your small intestine.) People with diabetes need to be very careful about fish oil supplements. The capsules can raise your blood sugar.

Old-fashioned codfish liver oil isn't a good way to get your fish oil. Aside from the truly objectionable flavor, cod-fish liver oil is very high in vitamins A and D. It's possible to overdose on these vitamins, so it's best to avoid codfish liver oil.

Because fish oil thins your blood slightly, it also may cause excess bleeding and could raise your risk of a hemor-rhagic stroke slightly. If you have a bleeding disorder or take any sort of blood-thinning medication, such as aspirin or Coumadin® (warfarin), fish oil could cause problems. Fortu-nately, just eating fish a couple of times a week is very un-likely to have an effect on your bleeding time.

The evidence points to getting your fish oil from fish, not supplements, whenever possible. If you'd like to try fish oil supplements to treat a specific health problem, talk to your doctor first.

When deciding which kind of fish to eat, remember that

freshwater fish and many of the most popular kinds of flaky
white fish, such as flounder, are low in omega-3 fatty acids.
Also, because these fish are often breaded and fried or are
used in prepared foods such as fish sticks, they are high in
trans fats. To get the most benefit from eating fish, select
oilier fish such as salmon, tuna, anchovies, sardines, eel,
herring, mullet, or mackerel. Steam, bake, or broil your fish,
but don't fry it—the high temperatures of frying destroy the
omega-3 oils.

FLAXSEED OIL

The richest vegetable source of the omega-3 fatty acid alpha
linolenic acid (LNA) is flaxseed oil. In fact, flaxseed oil has
about twice the LNA as fish oil. Flaxseeds and flaxseed oil
are high in LNA and fiber and also contain lignans, a type of
insoluble fiber that may play a role in preventing heart disease by reducing the risk of blood clots.

A number of studies have looked at the benefits of
flaxseed oil for a wide variety of health problems. Like fish
oil, flaxseed oil has been shown to help reduce high total
cholesterol and high LDL cholesterol and to have a beneficial effect on heart rhythm. Flaxseed oil also may help your
arteries be more flexible, which can help prevent heart attacks and angina.[31]

Flaxseed oil also has been studied for treating rheumatoid arthritis and other inflammatory conditions. The idea
behind the research is that LNA promotes the production of
anti-inflammatory prostaglandins, which in turn help reduce
pain and swelling. The advantage of flaxseed oil is that it is
much easier to tolerate than fish oil—no digestive upsets and
no fishy smell. Unfortunately, there's just not a lot of solid
research to show that flaxseed oil really works for other conditions, such as psoriasis and high blood pressure. On the
other hand, raising your LNA level has been shown to be a
good thing in general, which explains why flaxseed oil is

now one of the most popular supplements sold in health food stores.

Flaxseed oil has a light yellow color and a slightly buttery, mild flavor. The oil breaks down quickly when it's heated, so flaxseed oil shouldn't be used for cooking. It makes an excellent salad oil, however, and it also can be used instead of butter as a topping on vegetables. If you want to add flaxseed oil to your diet, you can buy it in capsules or as bottled oil. In either case, select an organically grown, cold-pressed product that has been kept under refrigeration. Flaxseed oil oxidizes easily. Store the container in a cold, dark place—the refrigerator is ideal—and use the oil quickly. If it develops an off taste, it probably has gone rancid and should be discarded.

Crushed flaxseeds are an excellent source of dietary fiber in addition to the LNA they contain. An alternative to using flaxseed oil is to use the crushed seeds themselves. They make a great crunchy topping for breakfast cereal or yogurt; they also can be mixed in with applesauce or juice.

OMEGA-6 FATTY ACIDS

Because your body uses omega-6 fatty acids to manufacture a series of prostaglandins that are associated with inflammatory processes such as swelling, eating less of them and more omega-3s may help relieve some health problems. Some health problems, however, may be helped by eating more omega-6s. In particular, a type of omega-6 fatty acid called gamma linolenic acid (GLA) may help relieve diabetic neuropathy (a painful nerve condition), premenstrual syndrome, eczema, and rheumatoid arthritis.

Although GLA has been extensively studied for these and other conditions, the evidence in its favor is good only for diabetic neuropathy and for rheumatoid arthritis. For diabetic neuropathy, the doses need to be fairly high—around 6 grams a day.[32] The optimal dose for rheumatoid arthritis isn't known, but one study showed that patients improved when they took 2 grams a day.[33] The most popular use of GLA is for treating premenstrual syndrome. Although some women swear it helps, unfortunately, the scientific evidence doesn't hold up very well.[34]

The main source of GLA is the tiny seeds of the evening primrose plant; GLA also is made from borage and black currant. It's usually sold in capsules. In general, GLA is quite safe, with negligible side effects and no known drug interactions. Even so, if you'd like to try it to treat diabetic neuropathy or rheumatoid arthritis, talk to your doctor first.

SMARTER BABIES

Everyone, not just adults, needs essential fatty acids, but infants and toddlers need them even more because they're growing so fast. That's why every medical authority strongly advises against limiting dietary fat for small children.

Human breast milk is very high in essential fatty acids, including DHA and arachidonic acid (AA). Although adults can manufacture both DHA and AA from other omega-3 fatty acids, babies can't do this as well—they make only small amounts of these fatty acids and rely on getting more from breast milk. DHA and AA are crucial for helping a newborn's rapidly growing brain and eyes develop properly; they're even more important for premature babies, who can't manufacture them at all.

A number of very solid studies have shown the importance of DHA and AA for infant development. To look at just two recent ones, a study in 2000 showed that infants fed a baby formula supplemented with DHA and AA performed better on tests of mental development than infants who got just regular formula. Not only did the supplemented babies do better, the improvements were large. Of the babies who got the DHA/AA formula, 26 percent scored over 115 on a standard IQ test, as compared to only 5 percent of those on the unenriched formula.[35] Another recent study showed that babies born to women who ate a lot of fatty fish, which is high in DHA, during pregnancy had better visual development by age three.[36]

The value of DHA and AA as additions to infant formula is widely accepted in Europe, Japan, and nearly sixty countries worldwide; it also is endorsed by the World Health Organization. The United States is just catching on, however. In 2001 the FDA finally approved adding DHA and AA to infant formula.

Chapter Eight
EATING THE GOOD FATS

For centuries the people of the Mediterranean countries have been living proof that a diet with no trans fats, little saturated fat, and lots of olive oil and polyunsaturated fat contributes to a long, healthy life.

EAT LIKE A GREEK

Starting in the late 1950s, the famous Seven Countries Study looked at the dietary fat intakes of people in the United States and different parts of Europe. This study was the first attempt to correlate diets high in saturated fat with high rates of heart disease. Whether the Seven Countries Study really proved that part of the hypothesis or not, it showed something else that in the long run is perhaps much more interesting. Of all the groups in the seven countries (Finland, Greece, Italy, Japan, the Netherlands, the United States, and Yugoslavia), the people of the Mediterranean island of Crete, off the southern coast of Greece, had the lowest rate of heart disease and among the highest rates of longevity. The people of Greece and southern Italy weren't far behind. Taken as a whole, in Greece in the early 1960s, there were 48 deaths from heart attacks per 100,000 men aged fifty to fifty-four. In the United States, there were 466 deaths per 100,000 men in the same age bracket. To put that another way, the death rate from heart attack in Greece was 90 percent lower. Among women in Greece, rates of breast cancer were much lower than among women in the United States. Throughout Greece, rates of all chronic diseases such as diabetes, heart disease, and cancer were much lower than in the United States, and Greek men had the highest life expectancy in the world.[1]

But according to the received low-fat wisdom, all those Greek people shouldn't have been anywhere near as healthy or long-lived, because they took in a whopping 40 percent of their daily calories from fat. American men who took in fat at that level were dropping dead from heart attacks, while Greek men were living healthy and very long lives—even though they didn't have access to the sophisticated medical care the American men got.

Why was there such a difference? Many factors come into this question, but one clear difference was in the type of fat. Greek men got 29 percent of their fat calories from monounsaturated fat—in other words, almost entirely from olive oil. They got only 8 percent from saturated fat and only 3 percent from polyunsaturated fat.[2]

In general, the traditional diet of people in Greece, Italy, and other countries in the Mediterranean region is high in fresh fruits and vegetables, olive oil, whole grains, low-fat dairy products, and fish. It's low in processed foods, sugar, trans fats, and red meat. And in general, the people who eat this diet are healthier than those who don't. Plenty of evidence now shows that even though these people take in well over 30 percent of their calories from fat, they're healthier than the people who eat the prudent, low-fat diet most American and European doctors now recommend.

The evidence in favor of eating a Mediterranean diet is so compelling that the International Task Force for Prevention of Coronary Heart Disease (sponsored by the World Heart Federation) issued an international consensus statement in 2000 endorsing it. Here's what the task force said:

There is increasing scientific evidence that there are positive health effects from diets which are high in fruits, vegetables, legumes, and whole grains, and which include fish, nuts and low-fat dairy products. Such diets need not be restricted in total fat as long as there is not an excess of calories, and emphasize predominantly vegetable oils that are low in saturated fat and partially-hydrogenated oils. The traditional Mediterranean Diet, whose principal source of fat is olive oil, encompasses these dietary characteristics.[3]

UNDERSTANDING THE MEDITERRANEAN DIET

There's no one Mediterranean diet—rather, there are food patterns found in some Mediterranean regions such as southern Italy in the 1960s. Broadly speaking, the Mediterranean diet has these characteristics:

- Plenty of plant food from fruits, vegetables, high-quality bread, potatoes, beans, nuts, and seeds.

- Fresh fruit daily instead of sugary desserts or sweets.

- Olive oil as the principal source of fat.

- Cheese, yogurt, and other low-fat dairy products daily in low to moderate amounts—but very little or no milk, cream, or butter.

- Fish and poultry in low to moderate amounts.

- No more than four eggs weekly.

- Red meat in low amounts.

• Wine in low to moderate amounts, normally with meals.

• Minimally processed, seasonally fresh, locally grown foods.

Coupled with the Mediterranean diet of the 1960s is the Mediterranean lifestyle of the period, which incorporated regular physical activity. Then as now, the combination of diet and exercise prevents obesity.

As the international consensus statement points out, "The Mediterranean style of eating describes a dietary pattern that is attractive for its famous palatability as well as for its health benefits."

SCIENTIFIC EVIDENCE

If you still need convincing about the merits of the Mediterranean diet, consider the results of the well-known Lyon Diet Heart Study. This long-term study conducted by scientists at INSERM, the French national research center, looked at 600 men and women who had just had their first heart attack. Half the group were told to eat a traditional Mediterranean diet; the other half were told to eat the prudent diet recommended by the American Heart Association. After a bit more than two years, the death rate from heart disease among the patients assigned to the Mediterranean diet was about 30 percent lower than the death rate in the prudent group. The chances of another, nonfatal heart attack also were much lower for the Mediterranean group, by at least 50 percent.[4]

What made the difference? According to the researchers, the difference was in the fat content of the diet. The patients on the Mediterranean diet got 30 percent of their calories from fat, of which 8 percent were from saturated fat; they ate about 200 mg of cholesterol daily. The prudent diet patients got 34 percent of their calories from fat, of which almost 12 percent came from saturated fat; they ate about 300 mg of cholesterol daily. Overall, the Mediterranean group ate slightly less total fat, saturated fat, and cholesterol but more olive oil and fish oil. To put it more simply, the fats the patients got from the olive oil, fish, whole grains, and green leafy vegetables had a protective effect.

What's particularly interesting about the first Lyon study is that the patients in the Mediterranean group had a better survival rate even though their blood lipids, blood pressure, and body weight were similar to the patients in the prudent diet group and even though the number of smokers in each group stayed the same.

The results of the Lyon Heart Study were confirmed by an additional study published in 1998. This time, the researchers showed not only that the Mediterranean diet prolonged the survival time of the heart patients, it also seemed to reduce their rate of cancer. Compared to the prudent diet group, the Mediterranean diet patients had a 56 percent lower risk of death from any cause and a 61 percent lower risk of death from cancer.[5]

The final report of the Lyon Diet Heart Study appeared in 1999. It showed that the heart-protective effects of the Mediterranean diet last for at least four years after a first heart attack. It also showed that patients on the Mediterranean diet continued to have a 50 to 70 percent lower risk of recurrent heart disease, such as angina or a second heart attack, and a much lower death rate.[6]

Not surprisingly, the American Heart Association has some objections to the Lyon Diet Heart Study. The AHA says the Lyon study isn't really a head-to-head comparison. The Mediterranean group worked closely with the researchers, while the prudent diet group were treated by their primary care physicians. The Mediterranean group may have stuck to their diet better, while the prudent dieters could have cheated. The AHA also would normally recommend less saturated fat than the prudent diet group ate. According to the AHA, if the prudent diet group had been following the lower-fat Step II diet, instead of the Step I diet, the disparity in the results wouldn't have been as large.

In light of the strong evidence, the cheater hypothesis and the Step I/Step II hypothesis don't hold up very well. The AHA is left with only one other main objection: Too much olive oil in the diet might cause obesity. Given that too many french fries made with deadly trans fats are a much more likely cause of obesity in the United States, this objection too is fairly feeble.

In fact, the AHA has recently recognized the importance of the Lyon results, stating that a Mediterranean-style Step I diet may help reduce the recurrent events in patients with heart disease. The new dietary guidelines actually incorporate some of the dietary evidence from the Lyon Heart Study. In particular, the Step I and Step II diets include more unsaturated fats and recommend eating fish twice a week.

It's also important to remember that even before the new AHA guidelines were issued, the Step I and Step II diets were a definite improvement over the typical American diet. When the diets of nearly 45,000 men were followed for eight years as part of the ongoing Physicians' Health Study, the benefits of the prudent diet were shown very clearly. The men who followed the basics of a prudent diet most closely—high intake of vegetables, fruits, legumes, whole grains, fish, and poultry—had one-third the risk of cardiovascular disease as the men who followed a typical American diet high in red meat, processed meat, refined grains, sweets and desserts, french fries, and high-fat dairy products. The men who followed the prudent diet most closely also were more likely to take multivitamin and vitamin E supplements and to exercise more; they were also less likely to be smokers. Even when these nondietary factors are taken into account, the prudent diet is clearly more healthful for your heart than the typical diet.[7]

BEYOND HEART HEALTH

The Mediterranean diet has gotten the most publicity for the way it helps your heart, especially if you've already had a heart attack, but there's a growing body of evidence that it helps the rest of you too.

One of the most interesting studies was recently released by the Seven Countries Study Research Group, which has been looking for more than 25 years at the diets of people in the original seven countries discussed above. The study looked at the relation between high blood pressure and death rates from coronary heart disease among men in different parts of the world. The results showed that men with slightly high blood pressure were more than three times as likely to die from heart disease in the United States and northern Europe as men with equally high blood pressure in Japan and Mediterranean southern Europe. Having high blood pressure still raised the relative risk of death for all the men, of course, but the absolute risk was lower for the Japanese and southern Mediterranean men.

The Seven Countries researchers don't claim that the Mediterranean diet or Japanese diet (which is very high in fish) alone is responsible for the difference in death rates, but they do point out that in addition to all the usual steps to lower blood pressure, like losing weight, quitting smoking, and taking medicine if necessary, changes in diet may play a very important role.[8]

The evidence for other health benefits of the Mediterranean diet is pretty solid as well. A study in 1998 backed up the finding in the original Seven Countries that women who ate a traditional Mediterranean diet had lower rates of breast cancer. The study looked again at over 66,000 women in Spain, Greece, and Italy, and found, as other studies have, that there was no statistical relation between breast cancer and the amount of saturated fat in the diet. The researchers found, however, that an increased consumption of monounsaturated fat (mostly olive oil) was associated with significantly *decreased* risk of breast cancer and consumption of polyunsaturated fat (mostly from margarine) with a significantly *increased* risk.[9]

To take just one more example of recent studies showing the benefits of the Mediterranean diet, a 1999 study in Italy suggests that olive oil helps prevent age-related memory loss. In a study of nearly 300 Italian senior citizens, the ones who ate the most olive oil were also the most protected against age-related cognitive decline.[10]

A DIFFERENT FOOD PYRAMID

If all the evidence in this chapter has convinced you to start eating the Mediterranean way, use the diet pyramid shown on page 92 as your guide.

This food pyramid was developed jointly in 1994 by the Oldways Preservation and Exchange Trust, the World Health Organization, and the Harvard School of Public Health. As you'll see, the Mediterranean pyramid differs considerably from the USDA pyramid shown on page 10. In addition to the very different food recommendations, the Mediterranean pyramid incorporates daily physical activity, recommends drinking six glasses of water daily, and suggests wine in moderation.

The Mediterranean pyramid is built on a solid foundation of high-quality plant foods. At the base are whole grains and potatoes; just above the base are fruits, vegetables, beans and peas, and nuts. Sharply unlike the USDA pyramid, which lumps all fats together at the very tip of the pyramids and says to use them sparingly, the next layer of the Mediterranean pyramid is olive oil. Above that is cheese and yogurt.

Animal foods such as fish, poultry, and eggs are in the narrower part of the pyramid, topped by sweets. At the tip of the Mediterranean pyramid is red meat, which should be eaten only occasionally.

The USDA pyramid specifies the number and size of

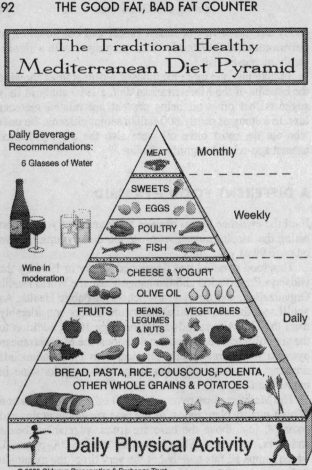

The Traditional Healthy Mediterranean Diet Pyramid

Daily Beverage Recommendations:

6 Glasses of Water

Wine in moderation

MEAT — Monthly

SWEETS

EGGS

POULTRY — Weekly

FISH

CHEESE & YOGURT

OLIVE OIL

FRUITS   BEANS, LEGUMES & NUTS   VEGETABLES — Daily

BREAD, PASTA, RICE, COUSCOUS, POLENTA, OTHER WHOLE GRAINS & POTATOES

Daily Physical Activity

© 2000 Oldways Preservation & Exchange Trust

servings for each food group. The Mediterranean pyramid shown here doesn't, although it does give an approximate idea of proportions and relative frequencies. That's because within each category there is an abundance of choices—and good health is always associated with a variety of foods selected according to individual preferences. The Mediterranean pyramid is suggestive, not prescriptive.

When planning meals around the Mediterranean pyramid, bear in mind that despite all the research, no one element of the diet is responsible for all the health benefits it gives. Olive oil, for instance, probably plays a big role, but so do all the many other different foods. Look at the diet as a flexible, delicious whole, not as a collection of disease-preventing elements, and enjoy the variety and flavor of the Mediterranean diet.

WHAT ABOUT WINE?

Historically, wine has always been a part of the traditional Mediterranean diet. A large body of evidence shows that moderate wine consumption (one to two glasses daily for men, one glass daily for women) is generally beneficial. Regularly drinking moderate amounts of red wine, for instance, can help raise your HDL cholesterol level. In fact, a study in Denmark showed that men and women who regularly drink wine not only have lower rates of death from heart disease and cancer, they have lower rates of death from any cause.[11] Alcohol of any sort, of course, should be restricted for children and teens, for people who can't limit their intake to moderate levels, for pregnant women, for people taking prescription and over-the-counter drugs, and for those planning to drive. That said, however, the evidence is strong in favor of choosing to enjoy a glass of wine with your Mediterranean-style dinner.

Wine is sometimes credited as the explanation for the so-called French paradox. In general, the French smoke more, exercise less, and drink more red wine than Americans do. Based on that, they should have higher rates of heart disease and some types of cancer, but in fact just the opposite is true: Their rates of these diseases are lower. A lot of researchers, many supported by the wine industry, are looking at the

French paradox. Many researchers believe that something in red wine—perhaps a compound called resveratrol—is responsible, but the studies are far from definitive. In general, though, they bear out the idea that wine, particularly red wine, has a beneficial effect, even if nobody is quite sure why.

THE IMPORTANCE OF EXERCISE

Improving your diet will almost certainly improve your health, but diet alone is not enough. To truly get the benefits of any diet—Mediterranean or otherwise—it must be accompanied by moderate physical activity on a daily basis. That doesn't mean joining an expensive health club and working out in aerobics class for an hour a day. Moderate physical activity can be as simple as spending half an hour going for a brisk walk or bike ride, working in the yard, or even doing housework. The important thing is to keep moving at a comfortable pace doing something that is both convenient and that you enjoy.

DASH FOR BETTER HEALTH

Since it began in the 1990s, the ongoing Dietary Approaches to Stop Hypertension (DASH) study, sponsored by the National Heart, Lung, and Blood Institute, has been showing that a diet high in fresh fruits and vegetables and low-fat dairy products and low in saturated fat can reduce high blood pressure. In fact, simply switching to this diet can lower mild high blood pressure in only eight weeks. It works just as well as prescription drugs—but without the cost and side effects.[12] The diet works even when if you don't lose weight or cut back on salt[13]—but if you do reduce salt intake, the DASH diet works even better.[14] More recent research has shown that the DASH diet also helps lower LDL cholesterol and raise

HDL cholesterol, although it doesn't seem to have any effect on triglyceride levels.[15] The DASH diet also seems to lower blood levels of homocysteine, an amino acid that is associated with a higher risk of heart disease and stroke.[16]

The DASH diet calls for eight to ten servings of fruits and vegetables daily, along with three cups of low-fat dairy food. The eating plan also calls for seven to eight servings daily of grains and grain products; two servings or less of meat, poultry, or fish; and just one daily serving of nuts, seeds, and beans and peas. Fats and oils are restricted to two to three servings a day. In general, serving sizes on the DASH diet vary between half a cup and one cup; a fat serving is counted as one tablespoon.

The DASH diet is low in fat, saturated fat, and cholesterol and rich in protein and fiber. It's also high in the minerals magnesium, potassium, and calcium. Eating the typical 2,000-calorie DASH diet provides about 4,700 milligrams of potassium, 500 milligrams of magnesium, and 1,240 milligrams of calcium—roughly twice as much as found in the typical American diet.

Are these nutrients the elements that help to lower your blood pressure? They all play an important role, especially the extra minerals, but it's almost impossible to separate the minerals from everything else in the foods on the diet. Fruits and vegetables in particular are high in vitamin C and many other complex nutrients as well as fiber and minerals.

Not only does the DASH diet work, it's so varied and gives you so much to eat that it's easy to stick with. While the diet still specifically recommends restricting dietary fat, it actually provides a lot of monounsaturated and polyunsaturated fats from dietary sources such as fish, whole grains, and green leafy vegetables. The DASH diet is lower (perhaps too low) in unsaturated fats than the Mediterranean diet, but beyond that the two diets have a lot in common. It's a hopeful sign that the medical establishment is starting to realize the crucial role of dietary fats for good health.

THE FAT COUNTER

The following fat count charts present the calories, total fat, saturated fat, monounsaturated fat, polyunsaturated fat, and cholesterol content of over 1,400 commonly eaten foods. The charts are based on information from the United States Department of Agriculture, food manufacturers, and fast-food restaurants.

The foods in the charts were selected for their overall fat content and because they are likely to contain trans fats. Because fresh fruits and vegetables don't contain much, if any, fat, for example, they have for the most part not been included. Processed vegetable products, however, which contain added fat (and often trans fats) from cheese, butter, and oils, have been listed.

The portion size given for each food item is based on the standard size used by nutritionists (usually 100 grams, or about 3 to 3.5 ounces) or on the portions provided by the manufacturer. In our age of the super-size meal, however, it's all too easy to eat more than the standard portion. When counting your calories and fat grams, look carefully at the portion size and be honest with yourself about how much you really ate.

Your goal is to get no more than 30 percent of your daily calories from fat. If you eat 2,000 calories a day, that works out to 600 calories from fat, or about 65 grams of fat. Of that, only 200 calories, or about 22 grams of fat, should come from saturated fat. Your cholesterol intake should be less than 300 mg a day. As few of your calories as possible should come from trans fat.

THE TRANS FAT TABLE

The separate table listing the trans fat count of selected foods that begins on page 113 is based on information from the United States Department of Agriculture and from the Harvard School of Public Health. Because food manufacturers are not legally required to list the trans fat content of their products, most don't provide it. In fact, this book may be the only place consumers can find this important information.

Until the new FDA labeling requirement goes into full effect, the trans fat content of a food will continue to be something of a mystery for consumers. Very few of the many thousands of food products that contain trans fats ever have been chemically analyzed to determine exactly how much trans fat is in each serving.

Some manufacturers have responded to public concern about trans fats by reducing how much they use. In future, more may do the same, so the trans fat contents listed here, while accurate, may well change in the future. The products in the trans fat chart are listed by their generic, not brand, names. In general, consumers should be able to make educated guesses about the brand names. A chocolate creme-filled sandwich cookie, for instance, can be nothing but an Oreo™.

In general, the more processed the food, the more likely it is to contain trans fats. Unprocessed foods such as fruits, vegetables, and grains contain no trans fats. Prepared potato products such as frozen french fries and home fries, however, are precooked in partially hydrogenated vegetable oil and are high in trans fats. Similarly, processed foods such as pasta contain no trans fats—but when pasta is processed further into an instant noodle product, trans fats are added. Prepared baked goods such as breads, cookies, crackers, snack cakes, doughnuts, cake, baking mixes, and pastries almost all contain trans fats. So do virtually all chip-type snacks. There are so many of these products—more than 6,590 different cookies are on the market—that it is impossible to list them all. To get a good idea of the fat content, representative brands are listed. Similar products are likely to have similar fat content.

HOW TO USE THE CHARTS

The fat counts are given in grams per portion; cholesterol is given in milligrams per portion. If the fat amount is left blank, it is usually because the manufacturer does not provide the information. When there is no amount given for the polyunsaturated fat content of a food, for example, this does not necessarily mean the product has none. When a product is known to contain none of a particular type of fat, this is indicated by 0.0. Remember that only animal products, such as milk, meat, poultry, and eggs, contain cholesterol.

ABBREVIATIONS

Use this key to understand the abbreviations in the tables:

chol	cholesterol
g	gram(s)
mg	milligram(s)
MUFA	monounsaturated fat
oz	ounce
PUFA	polyunsaturated fat
SFA	saturated fat
T	tablespoon
t	teaspoon
TFA	trans fat

Food	portion	calories	FAT	SFA	MUFA	FUFA	chol
FROZEN ENTREES							
beef, sliced, Banquet	1 entree	70	2.0	1.0			25
beef oriental, Lean Cuisine	1 entree	270	8.0	2.0		0.0	45
beef stew, Stouffers	1 entree	129	6.8				28
beef stroganoff, Stouffers	1 entree	159	10.2				45
burrito, beef and bean, Patio	1 entree	280	7.0	3.0			15
burrito, beef and cheese, Patio	1 entree	270	5.0	2.5			5
burrito, chicken, Patio	1 entree	260	4.0	1.5			15
cabbage, stuffed, with beef, Stouffers	1 entree	97	4.3				14
cannelloni, cheese, Stouffers	1 entree	172	8.3				20
chicken, glazed, Healthy Choice	1 entree	210	2.0	0.0			30
chicken, glazed, Lean Cuisine	1 entree	270	8.0	1.0		4.0	60
chicken cacciatore, Lean Cuisine	1 entree	280	10.0	1.0		2.0	45
chicken kiev, Le Menu	1 entree	491	31.6				
chicken marsala, Healthy Choice	1 entree	230	1.5	0.5			30
chicken marsala, Lean Cuisine	1 entree	190	5.0	1.0		1.0	75
chicken oriental, Lean Cuisine	1 entree	240	6.0	1.0		2.0	100
chicken parmesan, Lean Cuisine	1 entree	250	8.0	2.0		2.0	70
chicken primavera, Stouffers	1 entree	66	2.3				17

continued

Food	portion	calories	FAT	SFA	MUFA	FUFA	chol
chili, beef, Stouffers	1 entree	111	6.6				26
chow mein, chicken Lean Cuisine	1 entree	250	5.0	1.0		1.0	30
egg rolls, chicken, Chun King	1 entree	170	5.0	2.5			10
egg rolls, pork, Chun King	1 entree	170	6.0	1.5			5
egg rolls, shrimp, Chun King	1 entree	150	4.0	0.5			10
enchilada, beef, Patio	1 entree	200	6.0	3.0			10
enchilada, cheese, Patio	1 entree	170	4.0	2.0			10
fettucini alfredo, Healthy Choice	1 entree	250	5.0	2.0			15
filet of fish florentine, Lean Cuisine	1 entree	240	9.0	2.0		2.0	100
lasagna, Banquet	1 entree	230	8.0	4.0			35
lasagna, Lean Cuisine	1 entree	280	8.0	3.0		0.0	70
linguini, clam sauce, Lean Cuisine	1 entree	260	7.0	1.0		2.0	30
macaroni and cheese, Banquet	1 entree	210	5.0	2.0			10
macaroni and cheese, Healthy Choice	1 entree	290	5.0	2.0			15
meatballs, Swedish, Healthy Choice	1 entree	280	9.0	2.5			60
meatloaf with gravy, Banquet	1 entree	160	10.0	4.5			35
pepper steak, beef, Stouffers	1 entree	86	4.4				19
pizza, cheese, Jeno's Crisp 'n Tasty	½ pizza	272	13.7				
pizza, cheese, John's	½ pizza	249	12.0				

Food	portion	calories	FAT	SFA	MUFA	FUFA	chol
pizza, cheese, Lean Cuisine	½ pizza	310	9.0	3.0		2.0	10
pizza, cheese, Pillsbury microwave	½ pizza	242	9.8				
pizza, pepperoni, Jeno's Crips 'n Tasty	½ pizza	284	15.1				
pizza, pepperoni, Lean Cuisine	½ pizza	340	12.0	4.0		2.0	25
pot pie, beef, Banquet	1 entree	330	15.0	7.0			25
pot pie, beef, Swanson	1 entree	364	19.0				
pot pie, chicken, Banquet	1 entree	350	18.0	7.0			40
pot pie, chicken, Swanson	1 entree	379	21.7				
pot pie, chicken, Tyson	1 entree	567	36.6	8.3	13.0	4.2	23
pot pie, turkey, Banquet	1 entree	370	20.0	8.0			45
pot pie, turkey, Swanson	1 entree	381	21.4				
ravioli, cheese, Healthy Choice	1 entree	260	5.0	2.5			20
ravioli, cheese, Swanson	1 entree	273	7.5				
salisbury steak, Banquet	1 entree	220	16.0	7.0			25
salisbury steak, Stouffers	1 entree	241	14.6				73
tortellini, beef, Stouffers	1 entree	238	8.3				83
tortellini, cheese, Stouffers	1 entree	268	10.9				77
turkey, with gravy, Banquet	1 entree	140	9.0	4.0			30

continued

Food	portion	calories	FAT	SFA	MUFA	FUFA	chol
turkey tetrazzini, Stouffers	1 entree	238	14.3				43
veal parmigiana, Le Menu	1 entree	174	5.5	2.7		0.6	97

ICE CREAM AND PUDDING

Food	portion	calories	FAT	SFA	MUFA	FUFA	chol
banana pudding, from mix	½ cup	157	4.2	2.6	1.2	0.2	17
butterscotch pudding, Swiss Miss	4 oz	156	5.6	1.4			1
chocolate mousse	½ cup	446	32.9	18.5	10.3	1.7	299
chocolate pudding, from mix	½ cup	158	4.8	3.0	1.4	0.2	17
chocolate pudding, Swiss Miss	4 oz	166	5.7	1.5		0.0	1
custard, from mix	½ cup	162	5.5	3.0	1.7	0.3	81
custard, Swiss Miss	4 oz	153	5.3	1.2			4
flan, from mix	½ cup	150	4.1	2.5	1.2	0.2	16
ice cream, butter pecan, Häagen-Dazs	qq	236	13.9				
ice cream, chocolate	qq	143	7.3	4.5	2.1	0.3	22
ice cream, strawberry	qq	127	5.5	3.4			19
ice cream bar, chocolate, Häagen-Dazs	1 bar	361	24.7				
ice cream bar, vanilla, Häagen-Dazs	1 bar	332	22.6				
lemon pudding, from mix	½ cup	169	4.3	2.6	1.2	0.2	16
lemon pudding, Snack Pack	3.5 oz	124	3.1	0.9			0
pudding snacks, Jell-O	4 oz	159	5.1	1.9			0
rice pudding, from mix	½ oz	176	4.0	2.5	1.2	0.2	16
rice pudding, ready-to-eat	5 oz	231	10.6	1.7	4.6	4.0	1

Food	portion	calories	FAT	SFA	MUFA	FUFA	chol
tapioca pudding, from mix	½ cup	161	4.1	2.5	1.2	0.2	17
tapioca pudding, Snack Pack	3.5 oz	125	3.9	1.6			1
vanilla pudding, from mix	½ cup	155	4.2	2.6	1.2	0.2	17
vanilla pudding, Snack Pack	3.5 oz	135	4.9	1.3		1.0	1
yogurt, frozen	½ cup	115	4.3	2.6	1.3	0.2	4

MEATS

BEEF

Food	portion	calories	FAT	SFA	MUFA	FUFA	chol
brisket, braised	3.5 oz	291	19.5	7.5	8.7	0.7	93
chuck roast	3.5 oz	363	27.8	11.1	12.0	1.0	103
corned beef	3.5 oz	251	19.0	6.3	9.2	0.7	98
flank steak, braised	3.5 oz	263	16.4	6.9	6.9	0.5	72
ground, extra lean, broiled	3.5 oz	256	16.3	6.4	7.2	0.6	84
ground, lean, broiled	3.5 oz	272	18.5	7.3	8.1	0.7	87
ground, regular, broiled	3.5 oz	289	20.7	8.1	9.1	0.8	90
liver, braised	3.5 oz	161	4.9	1.9	0.7	1.1	389
pot roast, chuck	3.5 oz	348	25.8	10.2	11.1	1.0	99
round, bottom, roasted	3.5 oz	260	16.4	6.2	7.2	0.6	80
round, eye of, roasted	3.5 oz	241	14.1	5.5	6.1	0.5	72
round, top, broiled	3.5 oz	215	8.9	3.1	3.5	0.4	84
short ribs, braised	3.5 oz	471	42.0	17.8	18.9	1.5	94
steak, porterhouse	3.5 oz	327	25.6	9.9	11.3	0.9	75
steak, sirloin	3.5 oz	229	11.6	4.6	5.0	0.5	89

continued

Food	portion	calories	FAT	SFA	MUFA	FUFA	chol
steak, T-bone	3.5 oz	309	23.3	9.1	10.2	0.8	67
steak, tenderloin	3.5 oz	304	21.8	8.6	8.9	0.8	86
LAMB							
chop, loin	3.5 oz	316	23.1	9.8	9.7	1.7	100
chop, rib	3.5 oz	361	29.6	12.7	12.1	2.4	99
chop, shoulder	3.5 oz	281	19.6	8.4	8.0	1.6	96
leg, roasted	3.5 oz	225	12.4	5.1	5.3	0.9	90
LUNCHEON MEATS							
bologna, beef	1 slice	72	6.6	2.8	3.2	0.3	13
bologna, beef and pork	1 slice	73	6.5	2.5	3.1	0.6	13
bratwurst, pork, cooked	1 link	256	22.0	7.9	10.4	2.3	51
braunschweiger	1 slice	65	5.8	2.0	2.7	0.7	28
frankfurter, beef	1 frank	180	16.2	6.9	7.8	0.8	35
frankfurter, beef and pork	1 frank	182	16.6	6.1	7.8	1.6	28
frankfurter, turkey	1 frank	102	8.0	2.7	2.5	2.3	48
ham, baked	2 slices	47	1.2	0.4	0.6	0.1	24
olive loaf	1 slice	66	4.6	1.6	2.2	0.5	11
salami, beef	1 slice	60	4.8	2.1	2.2	0.2	15
salami, cotto	2 slices	93	7.1	3.1	3.2	0.4	38
salami, hard	1 slice	41	3.4	1.2	1.6	0.4	8
smoked link sausage, beef	1 link	128	11.5	4.8	5.4	0.4	27
smoked link sausage, pork	1 link	265	21.6	7.7	10.0	2.6	46
turkey breast	1 slice	23	0.3	0.1	0.1	0.1	9
vienna sausage	1 sausage	45	4.0	1.5	2.0	0.3	8
PORK							
bacon	2 slices	70	5.8	2.0	2.9	0.7	15
bacon, Canadian style	2 slices	67	4.0	1.3	1.9	0.4	27

Food	portion	calories	FAT	SFA	MUFA	FUFA	chol
chop, center rib, broiled	3.5 oz	260	15.8	5.8	7.0	1.2	82
chop, loin, broiled	3.5 oz	240	13.1	4.8	5.9	1.0	82
ham, cooked canned	3.5 oz	190	13.0	4.3	6.2	1.5	39
loin roast	3.5 oz	240	13.1	4.8	5.9	1.0	82
picnic, roasted	3.5 oz	280	21.4	7.7	10.1	2.3	58
sausage, fresh	1 link	48	4.1	1.4	1.8	0.5	11
VEAL							
chop, loin, braised	3.5 oz	284	17.2	6.7	6.7	1.2	118
ground, broiled	3.5 oz	172	7.6	3.0	2.8	0.6	103
liver, braised	3.5 oz	165	6.9	2.6	1.5	1.1	561
rib, roasted	3.5 oz	251	12.5	5.0	4.7	0.9	139
stew, braised	3.5 oz	188	4.3	1.3	1.4	0.5	145

MILK AND YOGURT

Food	portion	calories	FAT	SFA	MUFA	FUFA	chol
MILK							
buttermilk, cultured	8 oz	99	2.2	1.3	0.6	0.1	9
chocolate, whole	8 oz	208	8.5	5.3	2.5	0.3	31
cocoa, from mix	6 oz	103	1.2	0.7	0.4	0.0	2
condensed, sweetened	1 oz	122	3.3	2.1	0.9	0.1	13
eggnog, no alcohol	8 oz	342	19.0	11.3	5.7	0.9	149
evaporated, canned	1 oz	43	2.4	1.5	0.7	0.1	9
instant breakfast, chocolate, Carnation	8 oz	130	1.0				2
instant breakfast, chocolate, Pillsbury	8 oz	130	0.5				
lowfat, 1%	8 oz	102	2.6	1.6	0.7	0.1	10
lowfat, 2%	8 oz	1221	4.7	2.9	1.4	0.2	18
malted milk	8 oz	236	9.8	6.0	2.8	0.6	37
nonfat	8 oz	86	0.4	0.3	0.1	0.0	4

continued

Food	portion	calories	FAT	SFA	MUFA	FUFA	chol
soy milk	8 oz	79	4.6	0.5	0.8	2.0	0
whole	8 oz	157	8.9	5.6	2.6	0.3	35
YOGURT							
low fat, plain	8 oz	130	3.0	2.0			20
nonfat, plain	8 oz	130	0.0	0.0	0.0	0.0	10
whole, plain	8 oz	139	7.4	4.8	2.0	0.2	29
NUTS AND SEEDS							
almonds, dry roasted	1 oz	166	14.6	1.4	9.5	3.1	0
almonds, honey roasted	1 oz	169	14.1	1.0	7.8	3.6	0
almonds, oil roasted	1 oz	173	16.1	1.5	10.5	3.4	0
cashews, dry roasted	1 oz	163	13.1	2.6	7.7	2.2	0
cashews, honey roasted	1 oz	150	13.0	3.0	7.0	3.0	0
cashews, oil roasted	1 oz	163	13.7	2.7	8.1	2.3	0
coconut, dried, sweetened, flaked	1 cup	361	23.8	21.1	1.0	0.3	0
hazelnuts (filberts), dry roasted	1 oz	188	18.8	1.4	14.7	1.8	0
macadamia nuts, dry roasted	1 oz	200	21.1	2.5	16.3	0.6	0
mixed nuts, dry roasted	1 oz	168	14.6	2.0	8.9	3.1	0
peanut butter, chunky	2 T	188	16.0	3.1	7.5	4.5	0
peanut butter, smooth	2 T	190	16.3	3.3	7.8	4.4	0
peanuts, dry roasted	1 oz	160	14.1	2.0	7.0	4.4	0
peanuts, honey roasted	1 oz	150	13.0	2.0	7.0	4.0	0
peanuts, oil roasted	1 oz	165	14.0	1.9	6.9	4.4	0
peanuts, Spanish	1 oz	150	13.0	3.0	6.0	4.0	0
pecans, dry roasted	1 oz	187	18.3	1.5	11.4	4.5	0
pecans, oil roasted	1 oz	194	20.2	1.6	12.6	5.0	0
pine nuts	1 oz	160	14.4	2.2	5.4	6.1	0

Food	portion	calories	FAT	SFA	MUFA	FUFA	chol
pistachios, dry roasted	1 oz	172	15.0	1.9	10.1	2.3	0
sesame butter (tahini)	1 T	89	8.1	1.1	3.0	3.5	0
sunflower seeds, dry roasted	1 oz	165	14.1	1.5	2.7	9.3	0
sunflower seeds, oil roasted	1 oz	174	16.3	1.7	3.1	10.8	0
walnuts, dried	1 oz	190	19.0	2.0	6.0	11.0	0

POULTRY

CHICKEN

Food	portion	calories	FAT	SFA	MUFA	FUFA	chol
breast, fried, no skin	½ breast	161	4.1	1.1	1.5	0.9	78
breast, roasted, no skin	½ breast	142	3.1	0.9	1.1	0.7	73
breast, fried, with skin	½ breast	218	8.7	2.4	3.4	1.9	87
breast, roasted, with skin	½ breast	193	7.6	2.1	3.0	1.6	82
drumstick, fried, with skin	1 drumstick	120	6.7	1.8	2.7	1.6	44
drumstick, roasted, no skin	1 drumstick	76	2.5	0.7	0.8	0.6	41
drumstick, roasted, with skin	1 drumstick	112	5.8	1.6	2.2	1.3	47
liver, braised	3.5 oz	157	5.5	1.8	1.3	0.9	631
thigh, fried, with skin	1 thigh	162	9.3	2.5	3.6	2.1	60
thigh, roasted, no skin	1 thigh	153	9.6	2.7	3.8	2.1	58
wing, fried, with skin	1 wing	103	7.1	1.9	2.8	1.6	26
wing, roasted, with skin	1 wing	99	6.6	1.9	2.6	1.4	29

continued

Food	portion	calories	FAT	SFA	MUFA	FUFA	chol
DUCK							
duck, roasted, no skin	3.5 oz	201	11.2	4.2	3.7	1.4	89
duck, roasted, with skin	3.5 oz	337	28.4	9.7	12.9	3.6	84
TURKEY							
bacon	1 slice	34	2.7	0.8	1.1	0.7	13
breast, roasted, no skin	3.5 oz	157	3.2	1.0	0.6	0.9	69
breast, roasted, with skin	3.5 oz	197	8.3	2.3	2.8	2.0	76
dark meat, roasted, no skin	3.5 oz	187	7.2	2.4	1.6	2.2	85
dark meat, roasted, with skin	3.5 oz	221	11.5	3.5	3.6	3.1	89
ground	3.5 oz	170	9.8	2.9	3.8	2.9	84
SNACK FOODS							
Bugles	1⅓ cups	150	7.0	6.0			0
Bugles, baked	1½ cups	130	3.5	0.5			0
Bugles, nacho	1⅓ cups	160	9.0	7.0			0
Bugles, ranch	1⅓ cups	160	9.0	8.0			0
cheese puff/twists	1 oz	157	9.8	1.9	5.7	1.3	1
Cheez Curls, Planters	1 oz	150	10.0	2.0	3.5	0.0	
Chex Mix	1 oz	119	4.8	1.5			0
Combos Pretzel Cheddar Snacks	1 oz	131	4.8				1
corn cakes	2 cakes	70	0.4	0.1	0.1	0.2	0
corn cakes, blueberry crunch, Quaker	1 cake	49	0.2	0.0	0.1	0.1	0
corn cakes, white cheddar, Quaker	1 cake	38	0.3	0.1	0.1	0.1	0
corn chips	1 oz	153	9.5	1.3	2.7	4.7	0
corn chips, barbecue	1 oz	148	9.3	1.3	2.7	4.6	0
popcorn, caramel	1 cup	151	4.5	1.3	1.0	1.6	2

Food	portion	calories	FAT	SFA	MUFA	FUFA	chol
popcorn, caramel, Fiddle Faddle	¼ cup	150	7.0	3.0			10
popcorn, cheese, Pop Secret	1 cup	30	2.0	0.5			0
popcorn, cheese, Redenbacher	2 T unpopped	169	13.0	2.9			0
popcorn, Pop Secret	1 cup	35	2.5	0.5			0
popcorn, Redenbacher	2 T unpopped	168	12.5	2.7			0
popcorn cakes	2 cakes	77	0.6	0.1	0.2	0.3	0
popcorn cakes, caramel, Quaker	1 cake	47	0.3	0.0	0.1	0.1	0
potato chips, plain	1 oz	152	9.8	3.1	2.8	3.5	0
potato chips, sour cream and onion	1 oz	151	9.6	2.5	1.7	4.9	2
potato crisps, Pringles	1 oz	160	11.0	3.0			0
pretzels	1 oz	108	1.0	0.2	0.4	0.3	0
pretzels, chocolate-coated	1 oz	128	4.7	2.2	1.5	0.6	0
rice cakes, banana nut, Quaker	1 cake	50	0.3	0.1	0.1	0.1	0
rice cakes, chocolate crunch, Quaker	1 cake	50	0.3	0.1	0.1	0.1	0
rice cakes, Quaker	1 cake	35	0.3	0.1	0.1	0.1	0
tortilla chips	1 oz	142	7.4	1.4	4.4	1.0	0
tortilla chips, nacho	1 oz	141	7.3	1.4	4.3	1.0	1
tortilla chips, ranch	1 oz	139	6.7	1.3	4.0	0.9	0
SOUP, PREPARED							
bean with bacon	½ cup	180	5.0	2.0			3
beef, chunky	½ cup	85	2.5	1.5	1.2	0.0	7
beef broth	½ cup	15	0.0	0.0	0.0	0.0	3
beef mushroom	½ cup	32	1.5	0.7	0.6	0.0	4

continued

Food	portion	calories	FAT	SFA	MUFA	FUFA	chol
beef noodle	½ cup	70	2.5	1.0			15
black bean	½ cup	120	2.0	0.5			0
broccoli, cream of	½ cup	100	6.0	2.5			3
broccoli cheese	½ cup	110	7.0	3.0			10
celery, cream of	½ cup	82	4.6	2.0	1.4	1.3	16
chicken, chunky	½ cup	84	3.3	1.0	1.5	0.7	15
chicken broth	½ cup	30	2.0	0.5			3
chicken noodle	½ cup	70	2.0	1.0			15
chicken rice	½ cup	70	2.5	1.0			3
clam chowder, Manhattan	½ cup	60	0.5	0.0			3
clam chowder, New England	½ cup	100	2.5	1.0			3
lentil	½ cup	65	0.4	0.1			0
lentil, ham	½ cup	70	1.4	0.6	0.7	0.1	4
minestrone	½ cup	100	2.0	0.5			0
mushroom, cream of	½ cup	110	7.0	2.5			3
mushroom barley	½ cup	36	1.1	0.2	0.5	0.4	0
onion	½ cup	29	0.9	0.1	0.4	0.4	0
pea, split, with ham	½ cup	180	3.5	2.0			3
tomato	½ cup	100	2.0	0.0			0
tomato bisque	½ cup	130	3.0	1.5			5
vegetable, beef	½ cup	80	2.0	1.0			10
vegetarian	½ cup	70	1.0	0.0			0
VEGETABLES							
avocado, California	½ raw	306	30.0	4.5	19.4	3.5	0
avocado, Florida	½ raw	340	27.0	5.3	14.8	4.5	0
beans, baked, Campbell's	½ cup	180	3.0	1.0			5
beans, refried, canned	½ cup	114	1.6	0.6	0.7	0.2	10
beans with pork, Campbell's	½ cup	130	2.0	0.5			5

Food	portion	calories	FAT	SFA	MUFA	FUFA	chol
beans with pork, Hunt's	½ cup	130	1.2	0.4			0
broccoli, frozen	½ cup	26	0.1	0.0	0.0	0.1	0
broccoli, frozen, butter sauce	½ cup	40	2.0			0.0	5
broccoli, frozen, cheese sauce	½ cup	116	6.2	1.9		0.9	6
brussels sprouts, frozen	½ cup	33	0.3	0.1	0.0	0.2	0
brussels sprouts, frozen, butter sauce	½ cup	40	1.0			0.0	5
brussels sprouts, frozen, cheese sauce	½ cup	113	5.6	1.7		0.9	5
cauliflower, frozen	½ cup	17	0.2	0.0	0.0	0.1	0
cauliflower, frozen, cheese sauce	½ cup	114	6.1	1.9		0.9	6
chickpea hummus	½ cup	210	10.4	1.5	4.3	3.9	0
corn, cream style, canned	½ cup	59	0.3	0.1	0.1	0.2	0
corn, kernels, canned	½ cup	66	0.8	0.1	0.2	0.4	0
eggplant, boiled	½ cup	13	0.1	0.0	0.0	0.0	0
eggplant, fried sticks	½ cup	240	12.3				
eggplant, parmigiana, frozen	½ cup	264	16.4				6
green beans, frozen	½ cup	19	0.1	0.0	0.0	0.1	0
green beans, almonds, frozen	½ cup	52	1.6	0.2		0.5	0
green beans, butter sauce, frozen	½ cup	52	2.8	0.8		0.0	5
lima beans, frozen	½ cup	85	0.3	0.1	0.0	0.1	0
lima beans, butter sauce, frozen	½ cup	100	3.0	1.0		0.0	5
onions, cream sauce, frozen	½ cup	100	5.9	1.2		1.1	1

continued

Food	portion	calories	FAT	SFA	MUFA	FUFA	chol
onion rings, frozen	7 rings	285	18.7	6.0	7.6	3.6	0
peas, frozen	½ cup	62	0.2	0.0	0.0	0.1	0
peas, cream sauce, frozen	½ cup	118	5.6	1.1		1.0	1
potato, cheddar cheese, frozen	1 potato	228	10.8	7.2	3.3	0.3	6
potato, skin	1 potato	220	0.2	0.1	0.0	0.1	0
potato puffs, frozen	½ cup	138	6.7	3.2	2.7	0.5	0
potatoes au gratin, frozen	½ cup	161	9.3	4.0	3.0	1.0	28
potatoes au gratin, mix	½ cup	127	5.6	3.5	1.6	0.2	21
potatoes, cottage fries, frozen	½ cup	109	4.1	1.9	1.7	0.3	0
potatoes, french fries, frozen	½ cup	167	9.4	3.0	5.7	0.7	0
potatoes, hash brown, frozen	½ cup	163	10.8	4.2	4.8	1.2	0
potatoes, mashed, flakes	½ cup	119	5.9	3.6	1.7	0.3	15
potatoes, scalloped, frozen	½ cup	98	3.5				8
potatoes, scalloped, mix	½ cup	127	5.9	3.6	1.7	0.3	15
potatoes, Tater Tots, frozen	½ cup	161	7.3	1.3	5.1	1.0	0
spinach, boiled	½ cup	21	0.2	0.0	0.0	0.1	0
spinach, creamed, frozen	½ cup	60	2.0	1.0			2
sweet potato, baked	1 sweet potato	117	0.1	0.0	0.0	0.1	0
sweet potato, mashed	½ cup	172	0.5	0.1	0.0	0.2	0
sweet potato, syrup, canned	½ cup	106	0.3	0.1	0.0	0.1	0
sweet potato, whipped, frozen	½ cup	139	5.5				16

Trans Fat Content of Selected Foods

Food	Trans fat content in mg/100 grams
baby food, vegetable beef dinner	0.15
bacon	0.53
bacon fat	0.79
beans, refried	0.01
beef	
ground	1.68
ground, lean	1.50
ground, extra lean	1.32
heart	0.31
roast	1.75
sirloin steak	0.95
beef fat (tallow)	8.14
biscuit	
buttermilk	3.18
buttermilk, Pillsbury	4.00
cornbread	1.65
KFC	4.00
plain, dry mix	2.67
plain, refrigerated	4.06
bologna, beef	1.52
bouillon cube	
beef	3.20
chicken	3.85
bread	
cracked-wheat	0.99
dark	0.08
rye	0.14
white	1.39
bread crumbs, plain	0.07
breakfast bars	2.01

continued

Food	Trans fat content in mg/100 grams
breakfast cereal	
corn and oat, sweetened	0.34
cornflakes	0.15
crisp rice, sweetened	0.84
wheat/bran flakes with fruit/oat clusters	0.19
wheat/bran flakes with raisins and nuts	0.87
brownie	2.23
bun, cinnamon, Cinnabon	6.00
burrito	
bean	0.06
meat and bean	0.41
butter	3.71
buttermilk	0.03
cake	
chocolate fudge	2.00
pound	5.43
snack	2.26
yellow with frosting	3.44
candy, milk chocolate	0.49
candy bar	
chocolate cookie with caramel	6.92
chocolate nougat with caramel	1.6
chocolate with nuts	0.20
cheese	
American	1.43
American, low-fat	0.32
cheddar	1.52
cottage	0.20
cottage, low-fat	0.03
cream	1.59
cream, low-fat	1.06
mozzarella	1.45
cheese, grilled sandwich	1.82

Food	Trans fat content in mg/100 grams
cheese spread	0.65
cheeseburger, fast food	0.97
cheesecake	
fudge	3.00
plain	0.56
chicken	
fried, generic	0.36
fried, KFC dinner	7.00
roasted, with skin	0.04
roasted, without skin	0.02
chicken fat	0.36
chicken nuggets	
generic	4.46
McDonald's 9-piece	3.00
chicken pot pie	
Boston Market	4.00
KFC	8.00
chicken sandwich, Burger King	2.00
chili with beans	0.40
chips	
corn	0.64
potato	0.88
potato, light	0.53
chocolate	
hot	0.08
instant hot	0.07
clam chowder	0.24
coleslaw	0.07
cookies	
chocolate chip	5.84
chocolate sandwich	6.28
fig bars	1.16

continued

Food	Trans fat content in mg/100 grams
vanilla sandwich	7.09
vanilla wafer	4.25
cornbread	1.27
crackers	
cheese	7.43
cheese sandwich, peanut butter	3.01
graham	2.61
Ritz	1.00
saltine	3.07
snack	8.41
Triscuits	2.00
wheat	5.34
cream	
heavy	1.70
light	0.89
whipped	1.02
custard	0.13
diet bar	
Slimfast	1.30
Slimfast Ultra	0.09
doughnut	
cake, Dunkin' Donuts	6.00
cake, plain	6.91
fried	4.02
frosted, Entenmann's	5.00
yeast	2.45
eggroll	0.09
enchilada	
beef and cheese	0.31
chicken	1.14
Ensure	0.02
fish	
fried fillet, generic	0.49

Food	Trans fat content in mg/100 grams
Red Lobster Admiral's Feast	22.00
sandwich, Burger King	3.00
sticks, generic	1.78
stick, Van de Kamp's	5.00
French toast	1.12
frosting	
chocolate, creamy	3.52
marble, creamy	3.62
vanilla, creamy	4.04
fruit rollups	0.53
granola bar	
chocolate chip	1.96
low-fat	0.15
plain	0.22
gravy, beef	0.04
ham	0.08
hamburger	
fast food	0.96
vegetarian	0.62
hot dog	
beef	1.40
chicken	0.07
fast food beef	1.16
turkey	0.06
hummus	0.02
ice cream	
no-fat	0.02
vanilla	0.44
ice cream sundae, hot fudge	0.42
instant breakfast, Carnation	0.07
lard	1.56
lasagna	0.42

continued

Food	Trans fat content in mg/100 grams
liver	
beef	0.66
chicken	0.02
macaroni and cheese	0.55
margarine	
Benecol 37% tub	0.08
Benecol 65% tub	0.22
Blue Bonnet 53% stick	0.41
Brummel & Brown tub	0.12
Canoleo 785 tub	0.48
Corn oil, 80%, generic	0.65
Fleischmann 78% stick	0.65
Fleischmann 31% tub	0.14
Fleischmann 67% tub	0.38
Fleischmann 70% whipped	0.31
I Can't Believe spray	0.00
I Can't Believe 43% stick	0.32
I Can't Believe 70% stick	0.90
I Can't Believe 36% tub	0.14
I Can't Believe 70% tub	0.12
Imperial 705 stick	0.77
Land o' Lakes 42% blend stick	0.09
Land o' Lakes 78% blend stick	0.63
Land o' Lakes 42% blend tub	0.06
Land o' Lakes 80% stick	0.63
Olivio 60% tub	0.27
Parkay 60% squeeze	0.02
Parkay spray	0.01
President's Choice 40% tub	0.26
President's Choice 70% tub	0.65
Promise no-fat	0.00
Promise non-fat squeeze	0.00
Promise 43% stick	0.15

Food	Trans fat content in mg/100 grams
Promise 57% stick	0.12
Promise 70% stick	0.55
Promise 36% tub	0.12
Promise Ultra 25%	0.11
Shedd's 48% tub	0.18
Smartbalance 67%	0.08
Smartbeat tub	0.08
Smart Squeeze	0.00
Soybean oil, stick, generic	0.62
Take Control 40% tub	0.14
mayonnaise	
diet	0.24
regular	3.40
meatballs	1.22
meatloaf	1.08
Met RX bar	0.42
milk	
chocolate	0.04
powdered	0.03
1%	0.04
2%	0.08
whole	0.15
milkshake	
chocolate, fast-food low-fat	0.06
vanilla, fast-food	0.12
vanilla, fast-food low-fat	0.07
muffin	
bran	0.27
corn	3.55
English	0.02
wheat	0.20
nachos	1.15

continued

Food	Trans fat content in mg/100 grams
oil, olive	0.75
onion rings, fast food	4.00
pancakes	
cornmeal	0.44
flour	0.02
pastry	
Danish	4.11
Danish, low-fat	1.34
Danish, McDonald's cheese	4.00
Danish, pecan	2.13
peanut butter	0.77
pepperoni	0.36
pie	
apple	3.35
apple, Entenmann's	3.00
pumpkin	1.47
pizza	0.38
popcorn	
microwave	7.65
microwave, low-fat	3.16
oil-popped	12.37
pork, loin	0.18
pork and beans	0.03
pork rinds	0.58
potato chips	1.77
potatoes	
french-fried, Arby's	3.00
french-fried, Burger King	6.33
french-fried, frozen	2.67
french-fried, Hardee's	4.00
french-fried, McDonald's	3.41
french-fried, Ore-Ida	2.00
french-fried, Wendy's	7.00

Food	Trans fat content in mg/100 grams
mashed	0.02
scalloped	0.16
tater tots, Ore-Ida	2.00
potato salad	0.08
pretzel	0.61
pudding	
chocolate	0.04
rice	0.11
tapioca	0.08
vanilla	0.14
rolls	
cinnamon	2.36
dinner	0.33
hamburger	1.29
salad dressing	
French	0.27
Italian	0.64
lo-cal	0.13
no-fat	0.01
oil and vinegar	0.37
ranch	3.71
sauce	
cream	1.53
fudge	2.30
sausage	
fresh pork	0.34
kielbasa	1.27
processed beef and pork	0.40
processed pork	0.09
scone, Starbuck's cholesterol-free blueberry	4.00
sherbet, orange	0.08

continued

Food	Trans fat content in mg/100 grams
shortening	
Crisco	17.56
generic	19.59
shrimp, fried	2.17
snack cakes, creme-filled	0.68
soup, vegetable beef	0.05
sour cream	1.36
taco, beef and cheese	0.72
taco shell	7.98
tamale, beef	0.36
toaster pastry, Pop-Tart	1.34
tomato sauce, marinara	0.27
tortilla, wheat	1.06
tortilla chips	4.12
tuna salad	0.06
turkey, roasted	0.02
turnover, cornmeal	0.28
vegetables, oriental	0.18
yogurt	
frozen	0.25
low-fat, fruit	0.04
low-fat, plain	0.07

NOTES

CHAPTER ONE

1. M.L. McCullough, D. Feskanich, M.J. Stampfer, B.A. Rosner, F.B. Hu, et al., "Adherence to the Dietary Guidelines for Americans and Risk of Major Chronic Disease in Women," *American Journal of Clinical Nutrition* 172 (2000): 1214–22; and M. McCullough, D. Feskanich, E.B. Rimm, E.L. Giovannucci, A. Ascherio, et al., "Adherence to the Dietary Guidelines for Americans and Risk of Major Chronic Disease in Men," *American Journal of Clinical Nutrition* 72 (2000): 1223–31.

CHAPTER TWO

1. M.W. Gillman, L.A. Cupples, B.E. Millen, R.C. Ellison, and P.A. Wolf, "Inverse Association of Dietary Fat with Development of Ischemic Stroke in Men," *Journal of the American Medical Association* 278 (1997): 2145–50.

2. M. Kivipelto, E.-L. Helkala, M.P. Laakso, et al., "Midlife Vascular Risk Factors and Alzheimer's Disease in Later Life: Longitudinal, Population-Based Study," *British Medical Journal* 322 (2001): 1447–51.

3. M.L. Stefanick et al., "Effects of Diet and Exercise in Men and Postmenopausal Women with Low Levels of HDL Cholesterol and High Levels of LDL Cholesterol," *New England Journal of Medicine* 339 (1998): 12–20.

4. AHA Conference Proceedings, "Summary of the Sci-

entific Conference on Dietary Fatty Acids and Cardiovascular Health," *Circulation* 103 (2001): 1034.

CHAPTER THREE

1. R. P. M. Mensink and M. B. Katan, "Effect of Dietary Trans Fatty Acids on High-Density and Low-Density Lipoprotein Cholesterol Levels in Health Subjects," *New England Journal of Medicine* 323 (1990): 439–45.

2. M. B. Katan, P. L. Zock, and R. P. Mensink, "Effects of Fats and Fatty Acids on Blood Lipids in Humans: An Overview," *American Journal of Clinical Nutrition* 60 (1994): 1017S–22S; and J. T. Judd, B. A. Clevidence, R. A. Muesing, J. Wittes, M. E. Sunkin, and J. J. Podczasy, "Dietary Trans Fatty Acids: Effect of Plasma Lipids and Lipoproteins on Healthy Men and Women," *American Journal of Clinical Nutrition* 59 (1994): 861–68.

3. J. M. Gaziano et al., "Fasting Triglycerides, High-Density Lipoprotein, and Risk of Myocardial Infarction," *Circulation* 96 (1977): 2520–25.

4. A. H. Lichtenstein, L. M. Ausman, S. M. Jalbert, and E. J. Schaefer, "Effects of Different Forms of Dietary Hydrogenated Fats on Serum Lipoprotein Cholesterol Levels," *New England Journal of Medicine* 340 (1999): 1933–40.

5. N. de Roos, M. L. Bots, and M. B. Katan, "Replacement of Dietary Saturated Fatty Acids by Trans Fatty Acids Lowers Serum HDL Cholesterol and Impairs Endothelial Function in Healthy Men and Women," *Arteriosclerosis and Thrombosis* 21 (2001): 1233.

6. A. Ascherio, C. H. Hennekens, J. E. Buring, C. Master, M. J. Stampfer, and W. C. Willett, "Trans Fatty Acids Intake and Risk of Myocardial Infarction," *Circulation* 89 (1994): 94–101.

7. W. C. Willett and A. Ascherio, "Trans Fatty Acids: Are the Effects Only Marginal," *American Journal of Public Health* 84 (1994): 722–24.

8. A. Ascherio, E. F. Rimm, E. L. Giovannucci, D. Spiegelman, M. J. Stampfer, and W. C. Willett, "Dietary Fat

and Risk of Coronary Heart Disease in Men: Cohort Follow-up Study in the United States," *British Medical Journal* 313 (1996): 84–90.

9. F. B. Hu, M. J. Stampfer, J. E. Manson, et al., "Dietary Fat Intake and the Risk of Coronary Heart Disease in Women," *New England Journal of Medicine* 337 (1997): 1491–99.

10. A. H. Lichtenstein, "Trans Fatty Acids, Plasma Lipid Levels, and Risk of Developing Cardiovascular Disease," *Circulation* 95 (1997): 2588–90.

11. A. Ascherio, M. B. Katan, and M. J. Stampfer, "Trans Fatty Acids and Coronary Heart Disease," *New England Journal of Medicine* 340 (1999): 1994–98.

12. F. A. Kummerow, Q. Zhou, and M. M. Mahfouz, "Effect of Trans Fatty Acids on Calcium Influx into Human Arterial Endothelial Cells," *American Journal of Clinical Nutrition* 70 (1999): 832–38.

13. J. Salmerón, F. B. Hu, J. E. Manson, M. J. Stampfer, G. A. Colditz, E. B. Rimm, and W. C. Willett, "Dietary Fat Intake and Risk of Type 2 Diabetes in Women," *American Journal of Clinical Nutrition* 73 (2001): 1019–26.

14. M. T. Clandinin and M. S. Wilke, "Do Trans Fatty Acids Increase the Incidence of Type 2 Diabetes?" *American Journal of Clinical Nutrition* 73 (2001): 1001–2.

15. L. Kohlmeier, N. Simonsen, P. van't Veer, et al., "Adipose Tissue Trans Fatty Acids and Breast Cancer in the European Community Multicenter Study on Antioxidants, Myocardial Infarction, and Breast Cancer," *Cancer Epidemiology, Biomarkers and Prevention* 6 (1997): 705–10.

16. L. Kohlmeier, "Biomarkers of Fatty Acid Exposure and Breast Cancer Risk," *American Journal of Clinical Nutrition* 66 (1997): 1548S–56S.

17. W. C. Willett, "Dietary Fat and Breast Cancer," *Journal of Toxicological Sciences*, 52 (1999): 127–46; and C. Ip, "Review of the Effects of Trans Fatty Acids, Oleic Acid, n-3 Polyunsaturated Fatty Acids, and Conjugated Linoleic Acid on Mammary Carcinogenesis in Animals," *American Journal of Clinical Nutrition* 66 (1997): 1523S–29S.

18. W. McKelvey, S. Greenland, and R.S. Sandler, "A Second Look at the Relation between Colorectal Adenomas and Consumption of Foods Containing Partially Hydrogenated Oil," *Epidemiology* 11 (2000): 469–73.

19. T. Dunder, L. Kuikka, J. Turtien, L. Räsänen, and M. Uhari, "Diet, Serum Fatty Acids, and Atopic Diseases in Childhood," *Allergy* 56 (2001): 425–28.

20. M. Haby et al., "Asthma in Preschool Children," *Thorax* 56 (2001): 589–95.

21. J.M. Seddon, B. Rosner, R.D. Sperduto, et al., "Dietary Fat and the Risk for Advanced Age-Related Macular Degeneration," *Archives of Ophthalmology* 119 (2001): 1191–99.

CHAPTER FOUR

1. J.H. Dwyer, M. Navab, K.M. Dwyer, K. Hassan, P. Sun, et al., "Oxygenated Carotenoid Lutein and Progression of Early Atherosclerosis. The Los Angeles Atherosclerosis Study," *Circulation* 103 (2001): 2922–27.

2. F.B. Hu, M.J. Stampfer, E.B. Rimm, J.E. Manson, A. Ascherio, et al., "A Prospective Study of Egg Consumption and Risk of Cardiovascular Disease in Men and Women," *Journal of the American Medical Association* 281 (1999): 1387–94.

3. J.T. Braaten, P.J. Wood, F.W. Scott, M.S. Wolynetz, et al., "Oat Beta-Glucan Reduces Blood Cholesterol Concentrations in Hypercholesterolemic Subjects," *European Journal of Clinical Nutrition* 48 (1994): 465–74.

4. E.B. Rimm, A. Ascherio, E. Giovannucci, D. Speigelman, M.J. Stampfer, and W.C. Willett, "Vegetable, Fruit, and Cereal Fiber Intake and Risk of Coronary Heart Disease among Men," *Journal of the American Medical Association* 275 (1996): 447–51.

5. A. Wolk, J.E. Manson, M.J. Stampfer, G.A. Colditz, F.B. Hu, et al., "Long-term Intake of Dietary Fiber and Decreased Risk of Coronary Heart Disease among Women,"

Journal of the American Medical Association 28 (1999): 1999–2004.

6. D. J. Jenkins, C. W. Kendall, D. G. Popovich, et al., "Effect of a Very-High-Fiber Vegetable, Fruit, and Nut Diet on Serum Lipids and Colonic Function," *Metabolism* 50 (2001): 494–503.

7. T. A. Miettien, P. Puska, H. Gylling, H. Vanhanen, and E. Vartiainen, "Reduction of Serum Cholesterol with Sitostanol-Ester Margarine in a Mildly Hypercholesterolemic Population," *New England Journal of Medicine* 333 (1995): 1308–12.

8. D. Ornish, S. E. Brown, L. W. Scherwitz, J. H. Billings, et al., "Can Lifestyle Changes Reverse Coronary Heart Disease? The Lifestyle Heart Trial," *Lancet* 336 (1990): 129–33.

9. D. Ornish, L. B. Scherwitz, J. H. Billings, S. E. Brown, K. L. Gould, et al., "Intensive Lifestyle Changes for Reversal of Coronary Heart Disease," *Journal of the American Medical Association* 280 (1998): 2001–7.

10. R. J. Barnard, S. C. DiLauro, and S. B. Inkeles, "Effects of Intensive Diet and Exercise Prevention in Patients Taking Cholesterol-lowering Drugs," *American Journal of Cardiology* 79 (1997): 1112–14.

CHAPTER FIVE

1. D. B. Allison, S. K. Egan, L. M. Barraj, C. Caughman, M. Infante, and J. T. Heimbach, "Estimated Intakes of Trans-Fatty Acids and Other Fatty Acids by the U.S. Population," *Journal of the American Dietary Association* 99 (1999): 166–74.

2. *Federal Register*, vol. 64, no. 221, November 17, 1999, p. 62765.

3. Cardiovascular Review Group, Committee on Medical Aspects of Food Policy, "Report on Health and Social Subjects, 46, Nutritional Aspects of Cardiovascular Disease," Department of Health, London, Her Majesty's Stationery Office, 1994, p. 10.

4. " 'Eat Your Vegetables' Means French Fries to American Kids," Reuters Health, September 10, 1999.

5. World Health Organization, Health Behaviors in School-Aged Children Study, January 2000.

6. E. Schlosser, *Fast Food Nation* (Boston: Houghton Mifflin, 2001), p. 115.

7. A. H. Mokdad, M. K. Serdula, W. H. Dietz, B. A. Bowman, J. S. Marks, and J. P. Koplan, "The Spread of the Obesity Epidemic in the United States, 1991–1998," *Journal of the American Medical Association* 282 (1999): 1519–22.

8. A. K. Kantu, "Consumption of Energy-Dense, Nutrient-Poor Foods by Adult Americans: Nutrition and Health Implications," *American Journal of Clinical Nutrition* 72 (2000): 929–36.

9. S. Mickle and A. Moshfegh, USDA Food Surveys Research Group CDC Report, August 2000; and C. Zizza, A. M. Siega-Riz, and B. M. Popkin, "Significant Increase in Young Adults' Snacking between 1977–1978 and 1994–1996 Represents a Cause for Concern," *Preventive Medicine* 32 (2001): 303–10.

10. A. Ascherio, M. B. Kata, and M. J. Stampfer, "Trans Fatty Acids and Coronary Heart Disease," *New England Journal of Medicine* 340 (1999): 1994–98.

11. M. W. Gillman, L. A. Cupples, D. Gagnon, B. E. Millen, R. C. Ellison, and W. P. Castelli, "Margarine Intake and Subsequent Coronary Heart Disease in Men," *Epidemiology* 8 (1997): 144–49.

12. P. L. Zock and M. B. Katan, "Butter, Margarine and Serum Lipoproteins," *Arterioclerosis* 131 (1997): 7–16.

13. A. Ascherio, M. B. Katan, and M. J. Stampfer, "Trans Fatty Acids and Coronary Heart Disease," *New England Journal of Medicine* 340 (1999): 1994–98.

14. M. A. Denke, B. Adams-Huet, and A. T. Nguyen, "Individual Cholesterol Variation in Response to a Margarine- or Butter-based Diet," *Journal of the American Medical Association* 284 (2000): 2740–47.

15. A. H. Lichtenstein, "Trans Fatty Acids, Plasma Lipid Levels, and Risk of Developing Cardiovascular Disease," *Circulation* 95 (1997): 2588–90.

CHAPTER SIX

1. A. Ness et al., "Milk, Coronary Heart Disease and Mortality," *Journal of Epidemiology and Community Health* 55 (2001): 379–82.

2. K. M. Koehler, D. J. Zorn, and C. Nardinelli, "Dietary Fatty Acids and Cardiovascular Health. Dietary Recommendations for Fatty Acids: Is There Ample Evidence?" Abstract presented at the American Heart Association meeting, June 5–6, 1999, Reston, Virginia.

3. American Heart Association, "Coronary Heart Disease and Angina Pectoris," scientific statement, 1998.

CHAPTER SEVEN

1. J. M. Martin-Moreno, W. C. Willett, L. Gorgojo, et al., "Dietary Fat, Olive Oil Intake and Breast Cancer Risk," *Internal Journal of Cancer* 58 (1994): 774–80; M. C. Landa, N. Frago, and A. Tres, "Diet and Risk of Breast Cancer in Spain," *European Journal of Cancer Prevention* 3 (1994): 313–20; A. Trichopoulou, K. Katsouyanni, S. Stuver, et al., "Consumption of Olive Oil and Specific Food Groups in Relation to Breast Cancer Risk in Greece," *Journal of the National Cancer Institute* 87 (1995): 110–16; and C. La Vecchia, N. Negri, S. Franceschi, A. Decarli, and L. Lipworth, "Olive Oil, Other Dietary Fats and Risk of Breast Cancer," *Cancer Causes and Control* 6 (1995): 545–50.

2. W. Wolk, R. Bergstrom, D. Hunter, W. Willett, H. Ljung, et al., "A Prospective Study of Association of Monounsaturated Fat and Other Types of Fat with Risk of Breast Cancer," *Archives of Internal Medicine* 158 (1998): 41–45.

3. M. Goldacre et al., "Olive Oil, Diet and Colorectal Cancer: An Ecological Study and an Hypothesis," *Journal of Epidemiology and Community Health* 54 (2000): 756–60.

4. A. Espino-Montoro, J. Lopez-Miranda, P. Castro, et al., "Monounsaturated Fatty Acid Enriched Diets Lower Plasma Insulin Levels and Blood Pressure in Healthy Young Men," *Nutrition, Metabolism and Cardiovascular Disease* 6 (1996): 147–54.

5. L. A. Ferrara, A. S. Raimondi, L. d'Episcopo, L. Guida, A. Della Russo, and T. Marotta, "Olive Oil and Reduced Need for Antihypertensive Medications," *Archives of Internal Medicine* 160 (2000): 837–42.

6. A. C. Arntzenius, D. Kromhout, J. D. Barth, J. H. Reiber, et al., "Diet Lipoproteins and the Progression of Coronary Atherosclerosis. The Leiden Intervention Trial," *New England Journal of Medicine* 312 (1985): 805–11.

7. F. B. Hu, M. J. Stampfer, J. E. Manson, E. B. Rimm, G. A. Colditz, et al., "Frequent Nut Consumption and Risk of Coronary Heart Disease in Women: Prospective Cohort Study," *British Medical Journal* 317 (1998): 1341–45.

8. P. M. Kris-Etherton, G. Zhao, A. E. Binkoski, S. M. Coval, and T. D. Etherton, "The Effects of Nuts on Coronary Heart Disease Risk," *Nutrition Review* 59 (2001): 103–11.

9. R. U. Almario, "Effects of Walnut Consumption on Plasma Fatty Acids and Lipoproteins in Combined Hyperlipedemia," *American Journal of Clinical Nutrition* 74 (2001): 72–79.

10. P. M. Kris-Etherton, "Polyunsaturated Fatty Acids in the Food Chain in the United States," *American Journal of Clinical Nutrition* 71 (2000): S179–88.

11. F. B. Hu, M. J. Stampfer, J. E. Manson, E. B. Rimm, A. Wolk, et al., "Dietary Intake of Alpha-linolenic Acid and Risk of Fatal Ischemic Heart Disease among Women," *American Journal of Clinical Nutrition* 69 (1999): 890–97.

12. H. O. Bang, J. Dyerberg, and N. Hjorne, "The Composition of Food Consumed by Greenland Eskimos," *Acta Medica Scandinavica* 2000 (1973): 69–73.

13. A. Ascherio, E. B. Rimm, M. J. Stampfer, E. L. Giovannucci, and W. C. Willett, "Dietary Intake of Marine n-3 Fatty Acids, Fish Intake, and the Risk of Coronary Disease

among Men," *New England Journal of Medicine* 332 (1995): 977–82.

14. N. J. Stone, "Fish Consumption, Fish Oil, Lipids, and Coronary Heart Disease," *Circulation* 94 (1996): 2337–40.

15. M. L. Burr, A. M. Fehily, J. F. Gilbert, S. Rogers, R. M. Holliday, et al., "Effects of Changes in Fat, Fish, and Fibre Intakes on Death and Myocardial Reinfarction: Diet and Reinfarction Trial (DART)," *Lancet* 2 (1989): 757–61.

16. "Dietary Supplementation with n-3 Polyunsaturated Fatty Acids and Vitamin E after Myocardial Infarction: Results of the GISSI-Prevenzione Trial. Gruppo Italiano per lo Studio della Sopravivenza nell'Infarto Miocardico," *Lancet* 354 (1999): 447–55.

17. G. E. McVeigh, G. M. Brannon, H. N. Cohn, S. M. Finkelstein, R. J. Hayres, and G. D. Johnston, "Fish Oil Improves Arterial Compliance in Non-Insulin-Dependent Diabetes Mellitus," *Arteriosclerosis and Thrombosis* 14 (1994): 1425–29.

18. J. F. P. Chin, A. P. Gust, P. J. Nestel, and A. M. Dart, "Marine Oils Dose-Dependently Inhibit Vasoconstriction of Forearm Resistance Vessels in Humans," *Hypertension* 21 (1993): 22–28.

19. D. S. Siscovick, T. E. Raghunathan, I. King, S. Weinmann, et al., "Dietary Intake and Cell Membrane Level of Long-Chain n-3 Polyunsaturated Fatty Acids and the Risk of Primary Cardiac Arrest," *Journal of the American Medical Association* 274 (1995): 1363–67.

20. M. L. Daviglus, J. Stamler, A. J. Orencia, et al., "Fish Consumption and the 30-Year Risk of Fatal Myocardial Infarction," *New England Journal of Medicine* 15 (1997): 1046–53.

21. C. M. Albert, C. H. Hennekens, C. J. O'Donnell, U. A. Ajani, V. J. Cary, W. C. Willett, et al., "Fish Consumption and Risk of Sudden Cardiac Death," *Journal of the American Medical Association* 279 (1998): 23–28.

22. D. Mozaffarian, D. S. Siscovick, et al., paper pre-

sented at the American Heart Association Conference, February 2001.

23. C. Deck and K. Radack, "Effects of Modest Doses of Omega-3 Fatty Acids on Lipids and Lipoproteins in Hypertriglyceridemic Subjects. A Randomized Controlled Trial," *Archives of Internal Medicine* 149 (1989): 1857–82; K.L. Radack, C.C. Deck, and G.A. Huster, "N-3 Fatty Acid Effects on Lipids, Lipoproteins, and Apolipoproteins at Very Low Doses: Results of a Randomized Controlled Trial in Hypertriglyceridemic Subjects," *American Journal of Clinical Nutrition* 51 (1990): 599–605.

24. K.D. Stark, E.J. Park, V.A. Maines, and B.J. Holub, "Effect of a Fish-Oil Concentrate on Serum Lipids in Postmenopausal Women Receiving and Not Receiving Hormone Replacement Therapy in a Placebo-Controlled, Double-Blind Trial," *American Journal of Clinical Nutrition* 72 (2000): 389–94.

25. H. Iso, K.M. Rexrode, M.J. Stampfer, J.E. Manson, G.A. Colditz, et al., "Intake of Fish and Omega-3 Fatty Acids and Risk of Stroke in Women," *Journal of the American Medical Association* 285 (2001): 304–12.

26. M.C. Morris, F. Sacks, and B. Rosner, "Does Fish Oil Lower Blood Pressure? A Meta-Analysis of Controlled Trials," *Circulation* 88 (1993): 523–33.

27. E. Fernandez, L. Chatenoud, C. La Vecchia, E. Negri, and S. Franceshi, "Fish Consumption and Cancer Risk," *American Journal of Clinical Nutrition* 70 (1999): 85–90.

28. A.G. Schuurman, P.A. ven den Brandt, E. Dorant, H.A. Garnts, and R.A. Goldbohm, "Association of Energy and Fat Intake with Prostate Carcinoma Risk: Results from The Netherlands Cohort Study," *Cancer* 86 (1999): 1019–27.

29. P. Terry, P. Lichtenstein, M. Peychting, A. Ahlbom, and A. Wolk, "Fatty Fish Consumption and Risk of Prostate Cancer," *Lancet* 357 (2001): 1764–66.

30. J.M. Kremer, "N-3 Fatty Acid Supplements in Rheumatoid Arthritis," *American Journal of Clinical Nutrition* 71 (2000): 349S–51S.

31. P. H. Nestel, S. E. Pomeroy, T. Sasahara, et al., "Arterial Compliance in Obese Subjects Is Improved with Dietary Plant n-3 Fatty Acid from Flaxseed Oil Despite Increased LDL Oxidizability," *Arteriosclerosis and Thrombosis* 17 (1997): 1163–70.

32. H. Keen et al., "Treatment of Diabetic Neuropathy with Gamma-Linolenic Acid. The Gamma-Linolenic Acid Multicenter Trial Group," *Diabetes Care* 16 (1993): 8–15.

33. R. B. Zurier et al., "Gamma-Linolenic Acid Treatment of Rheumatoid Arthritis. A Randomized, Placebo-Controlled Trial," *Arthritis and Rheumatism* 39 (1996): 1808–17.

34. D. Budeiri et al., "Is Evening Primrose Oil of Value in the Treatment of Premenstrual Syndrome?" *Controlled Clinical Trials* 17 (1996): 60–68.

35. E. E. Birch, S. Garfield, D. R. Hoffman, R. Uauy, and D. G. Birch, "A Randomized Controlled Trial of Early Dietary Supply of Long-Chain Polyunsaturated Fatty Acids and Mental Development in Term Infants," *Developmental Medicine and Child Neurology* 42 (2000): 174–81.

36. S. J. Otto, A. C. van Houwelingen, A. Badart-Smook, and G. Hornstra, "Changes in the Maternal Essential Fatty Acid Profile during Early Pregnancy and the Relation of the Profile to Diet," *American Journal of Clinical Nutrition* 73 (2001): 302–7.

CHAPTER EIGHT

1. A. Keys et al., "Coronary Heart Disease in Seven Countries," *Circulation* 41 (Suppl. I) (1970): I-1—I-211.

2. D. Kromhout, A. Keys, C. Aravanis, et al., "Food Consumption Patterns in the 1960s in Seven Countries," *American Journal of Clinical Nutrition* 49 (1989): 889–94.

3. International Consensus Statement, International Conference on the Mediterranean Diet, Royal College of Physicians, London, January 13–14, 2000.

4. M. de Lorgeril, S. Renaud, N. Mamelle, et al., "Mediterranean Alpha-Linolenic Acid-Rich Diet in Sec-

ondary Prevention of Coronary Heart Disease," *Lancet* 343 (1994): 1454–59.

5. M. de Lorgeril, P. Salen, J.-L. Martin, et al., "Mediterranean Dietary Pattern in a Randomized Trial: Prolonged Survival and Possible Reduced Cancer Rate," *Archives of Internal Medicine* 158 (1998): 1181–87.

6. M. de Lorgeril, P. Salen, J.-L. Martin, et al., "Mediterranean Diet, Traditional Risk Factors, and the Rate of Cardiovascular Complications after Myocardial Infarction," *Circulation* 99 (1999): 779–85.

7. F. B. Hu et al., "Prospective Study of Major Dietary Patterns of Risk of Coronary Heart Disease in Men," *American Journal of Clinical Nutrition* 72 (2000): 912–21.

8. P. C. W. van den Hoogen et al., "The Relation between Blood Pressure and Mortality Due to Coronary Heart Disease among Men in Different Parts of the World," *New England Journal of Medicine* 342 (2000): 1–8.

9. A. Wolk, R. Bergstrom, D. Hunter, and W. Willett, "A Prospective Study of Association of Monounsaturated Fat and Other Types of Fat with Risk of Breast Cancer," *Archives of Internal Medicine* 158 (1998): 41–45.

10. V. Solfrizzi et al., "High Monounsaturated Fatty Acids Intake Protects against Age-Related Cognitive Decline," *Neurology* 52 (1999): 1563–69.

11. M. Gronbaek et al., "Type of Alcohol Consumed and Mortality from All Causes, Coronary Heart Disease, and Cancer," *Annals of Internal Medicine* 133 (2000): 411–19.

12. L. J. Appel et al., "A Clinical Trial of the Effects of Dietary Patterns on Blood Pressure. DASH Collaborative Research Group," *New England Journal of Medicine* 336 (1997): 1117–24.

13. L. P. Svetkey et al., "Effects of Dietary Patterns on Blood Pressure: Subgroup Analysis of the Dietary Approaches to Stop Hypertension (DASH) Randomized Clinical Trial," *Archives of Internal Medicine* 159 (1999): 285–93.

14. F. M. Sacks et al., "Effects on Blood Pressure of Reduced Dietary Sodium and the Dietary Approaches to Stop

Hypertension (DASH) Diet. DASH-Sodium Collaborative Research Group," *New England Journal of Medicine* 344 (2001): 3–10.

15. E. Obarzanke et al., "Effects on Blood Lipids of a Blood Pressure-Lowering Diet: The Dietary Approaches to Stop Hypertension (DASH) Trial," *American Journal of Clinical Nutrition* 74 (2001): 80–89.

16. L. J. Appel et al., "Effect of Dietary Patterns on Serum Homocysteine: Results of a Randomized, Controlled Feeding Study," *Circulation* 102 (2000): 852–57.

INDEX